RN's

Legally Speaking

How to Protect Your Patients and Your License

Edited by

Gayle Hacker Sullivan, RN, JD

Marianne Dekker Mattera

Medical Economics   Montvale, NJ

Library of Congress Catalog Number: 97-76588

ISBN: 1-56363-274-8

Manufactured in the United States of America

Bulk copy inquiries are invited. Contact the Trade Sales Department at 1-800-442-6657.

The information presented in this publication is based on research and consultation with legal and nursing experts. To the best of our knowledge, it represents current opinion and legal fact at the time of publication. It cannot be construed, however, as absolute and universal recommendations or as legal advice in any given situation. The authors and publisher disclaim responsibility for any adverse consequences that result from following the guidelines outlined here without first seeking legal advice, from undetected errors, or from misinterpretation by the reader.

Publishing staff: Marianne Dekker Mattera, editor; Jayne Jacobsen, assistant editor; Joanne Pearson, production associate, Robert Hartman, art director

Business staff: Paul Walsh, publisher; Marjorie Duffy, production director, Robin Bartlett, director of trade and direct marketing sales; Stephanie DiNardi and Steven Schweikhart, fulfillment managers.

Officers of Medical Economics: President and Chief Executive Officer: Curtis B. Allen; Vice President, Human Resources: Pamela M. Bilash; Vice President and Chief Information Officer: Steven M. Bressler; Vice President, Finance, and Chief Financial Officer: Thomas W. Ehardt; Executive Vice President and Chief Operating Officer: Rick Noble; Executive Vice President, Magazine Publishing: Thomas F. Rice; Senior Vice President, Operations: John R. Ware

About the Editors

Gayle Hacker Sullivan, RN, JD is founder and president of Quality Assurance Associates, Inc., a medical liability consulting firm in Fairfield, Conn. She conducts risk management seminars and loss control surveys for hospitals, nursing homes, home health agencies, and managed care organizations nationwide. Ms. Sullivan also produces risk management programs for satellite broadcast television and has received the International Teleconferencing Association award for Outstanding Achievement in direct broadcast satellite programs and services. She is a member of the adjunct faculty in the School of Nursing at Fairfield University, the American and New York Bar Associations, the American and Connecticut Nurses Associations, The American Association of Nurse Attorneys, Sigma Theta Tau, and the **RN** Editorial Board.

Marianne Dekker Mattera has been the Editor of **RN** since September 1990 and has been shaping the editorial direction there since 1983 when she joined the staff as Managing Editor. Ms. Mattera has received 13 Jesse H. Neal Awards—considered the Pulitzer Prize of specialized journalism—for editorial achievement. This spring she was presented with the Crain Award for significant career achievement. During her tenure, **RN** has been named a finalist in the National Magazine Award competition and has won three Regional Media Awards for Excellence in Nursing Journalism presented by Sigma Theta Tau. Ms. Mattera has lectured often to nurses, nursing students, educators, and professional journalists. She's been involved in writing and editing on legal topics since 1972.

Contents

Unit Three: Rights and Responsibilities

Unit Four: The Legal Process

Unit Five: Current Controversies

Unit Six: Malpractice Coverage

Appendices

Preface

This book has been a long time in the making. For years, **RN** has served as a consistent source of legal information for nurses. Our monthly department, Legally Speaking, has been on the top of readership surveys for more than a decade—readers turn to it without fail for pertinent, timely advice on safe nursing practice. It's also been singled out five times as a distinguished example of service journalism in prestigious publishing competitions.

Finally, we've collected, organized, and updated those valuable essays, written by well-known legal experts. After three of the units, you'll also find a Q&A section—questions from nurses just like you, and answers from some of the finest legal minds in the country. You'll find discussions of actual cases as well as legal theory and plenty of specific examples of situations you encounter every day. The unit on current controversies provides insight into the ramifications for nurses of such issues as assisted suicide, telemedicine, and managed care. One caveat, however: Laws change. The discussions here represent the law as it is today; it's up to you to keep tabs on what happens in your state tomorrow and all the tomorrows until our next edition.

We're convinced that this book is one of the most practical guides you'll ever find to the legal issues you face in day-to-day practice. And we're very excited to be bringing you this handy reference at long last.

Contributors

Linda M. Auton, RN, JD
Attorney in private practice
Abington, Mass.

Anna Blair, JD
General counsel
Helen Keller Hospital
Sheffield, Ala.

Penny Simpson Brooke,
RN, MSN, JD
Associate Professor and Assistant Dean
for Student Affairs
University of Utah College of Nursing
Salt Lake City

Patricia Carroll, RN,C, MS,
CEN, RRT
Educational Medical Consultants
Meriden, Conn.

Margaret Davino, RN, JD
Vice President of Legal Affairs
St. Vincent's Hospital
New York, N.Y.

Denise Liotta DeMarzo, RN, JD
Medical malpractice attorney
Clark, Gagliardi and Miller P.C.
White Plains, N.Y.

Susan J. Dycus, RN, JD
Attorney in private practice
Denver, Colo.

Tina Rae Eskreis-Nelson, RN,
BSN, JD
Asst. Attorney General
Office of the New York State Attorney
General and Adjunct Professor
New York University
New York, N.Y.

Judith A. Gic, RN, CRNA, JD
Attorney in private practice
New Orleans, La.

Linda J. Gobis, RN, FNP, JD
Kravit, Gass & Weber
Milwaukee, Wis.

Phyllis Granade, JD
Law offices of Kilpatrick Stockton LLP
Atlanta, Ga.

Paul Greve, JD
Vice President of Marketing
The Medical Protective Company
Ft. Wayne, Ind.

Jack Horsley, JD
Defense attorney
Craig & Craig
Mattoon, Illinois

Marie C. Infante, RN, JD, MS, MBA
Attorney in private practice
Washington, D.C.

Helen Lippman
Legal Editor, RN Magazine

Anne Maltz, RN, JD
General Counsel
MagnaCare
Garden City, N.Y.

Donna Lee Mantel, RN, JD
Certified civil trial attorney
Davis, Saperstein & Salomon
Teaneck, N.J.

Sue Masoorli, RN
President, Perivascular Nurse
Consultants, Inc.
Rockledge, Pa.

Donna Moniz, RN, JD
Johnson, Graffe, Keay & Moniz
Seattle, Wash.

Marilyn Pesto, RN, JD
Office of Corporate Counsel
Truman Medical Center
Kansas City, Mo.

Juanita Reigle, RN, MSN, CCRN
Assistant Professor of Nursing
University of Virginia School of
Nursing
Charlottesville, Va.

Mel Rutherford, JD
Vice President of Legal Services
Children's Hospital Medical Center
Cincinnati, Ohio

Mary Ann Shea, RN, JD
Midwest Medical/Legal Services
St. Louis, Mo.

Joanne P. Sheehan, RN, BSN, JD
Principal in the firm
of Friedman Mellitz & Newman P.C.
Fairfield, Conn.

Andrea Sloan, RN, JD
Attorney in private practice
McLean, Va.

Gayle Hacker Sullivan, RN, JD
President,
Quality Assurance Associates, Inc.
Fairfield, Conn.

Morna L. Sweeney, RN, JD
Medical malpractice
and product liability attorney
Porzio, Bromberg & Newman P.C.
Morristown, N.J.

David A. Tammelleo, Sr., JD
Attorney in private practice
Providence, R.I.

Stephanie E. Trudeau, JD
Partner in the firm of Ulmer & Berne LLP
Cleveland, Ohio

Angela M. Viera, RN, JD
Associate General Counsel and
Associate Director of Risk Management
New England Medical
Center Hospitals, Inc.
Boston, Mass.

Suzanne Wolfe, MA
Legal Editor, RN Magazine

Introduction

In the good old days, lawsuits were reserved for major disasters, and malpractice suits were rare. Today we live in the age of litigation: Everybody sues everybody else. A guest who's had too much to drink at a party and gets into a car accident on the way home sues his host for serving him more liquor than he could handle. A patron who slips on the ice in front of a store sues the merchant for not cleaning the sidewalk properly. And an increasing number of patients sue health care facilities, doctors, and nurses over insignificant injuries and minor mishaps.

What's the best way to protect yourself from a malpractice suit? Well, in the liability arena, the reverse of the old maxim is true: The best defense is a good offense. Aside from practicing exemplary nursing always, the best thing you can do to forestall a malpractice suit is to build a good rapport with your patients. In fact, the quality of the relationship between a patient and his caregiver is sometimes a better predictor of whether he files suit than the extent of his injury. People who feel they have been treated well tend to be more forgiving than those who feel they have been ignored or mistreated by their caregivers.

That being said, there are certain types of patients who are considered "suit-prone." If you approach their care aggressively, heading off complaints before they're lodged, there's a good chance you'll never wind up in court.

How do you recognize a "suit-prone" patient? Many of them are openly angry even before an incident or injury occurs. They gripe about everything: You take too long to answer his call bell, you don't do enough to alleviate her pain, or you expect too much of him. Or they refuse to comply with treatment for no good reason. Their hostility may reflect their own inner turmoil or their dissatisfaction with the quality of the care they receive.

Other types of suit-prone patients aren't as easy to spot. The patient who's withdrawn, sullen, or seemingly helpless, for instance, is easy to overlook. But he may be as depressed, angry, or fearful as a more combative patient and equally in need of attention. Those who have unrealistic expectations—like the cataract surgery patient who doesn't realize that it could take weeks for her vision to be fully restored—also fall into the suit-prone category. When a patient expects a perfect outcome to any procedure or treatment, the slightest complication may provoke the threat of a lawsuit.

Beware, too, of the very dependent patient. A woman may demand to be lifted out of bed for days after orthopedic surgery, for instance, despite her doctor's orders that she should be up and walking. A man may refuse to learn his wound-care protocol, expecting family members to do everything for him. Dependency is often the only manifestation of fear and hostility that some people exhibit.

Sometimes, it's not the patient but the family that fits the suit-prone profile. They may try to monopolize your time, complain that you are not doing enough for their loved one, or threaten to take their complaints over your head. Be just as wary of families like this as you are of angry patients—and pay just as much attention to them.

Unfortunately, nurses often avoid suit-prone patients, ignore them, or dismiss their complaints because they tend to be demanding and difficult to deal with. Thus, the very people who need more support and attention often end up getting less.

The next time you're confronted with a hostile or sullen patient—or family member—try defusing the anger instead of ignoring it. Acknowledge your patient's feelings: "You seem worried about your eye," you might say to someone who has just had reconstructive surgery and asks repeatedly for her ophthalmologist. "Would you like to tell me what's bothering you?" If she says Yes, listen intently. If she doesn't respond, assure her that you'll try to contact her physician, and suggest she call you whenever she'd like to discuss her concerns or complaints.

Always take problems seriously. Even when you're sure there's no basis for the worries expressed—if the family just finished talking to the attending physician, for example, or the surgeon just examined the patient's eye. Remember, the fear underlying the questions or complaints is real. Respond not only with reassurance but also with action. If you say you will speak to the physician, for instance, do so as quickly as possible.

To avoid surprises, spend extra time reviewing a procedure and its outcome with the preop patient, and additional time on patient teaching after surgery. Tell both the patient and his family members what will happen next. When is the doctor expected? About what time will you or another nurse be back? When is the next meal or next dose of pain medication scheduled? Having a timetable, even if it's not precise, can relieve the feeling that every minute is like an hour, and help restore a sense of control.

Anticipate needs. Ask the patient if there's anything you can do for her before you leave. Offer to meet with the family and the physician. Spend extra time with a troubled patient, too, even if it's only a few minutes. If your schedule doesn't permit that kind of attention, arrange for the chaplain, your hospital's patient representative, someone from social services, or even a volunteer to visit. You may want to call in the discharge planner earlier than usual as well.

Do everything possible to involve the patient in his own recovery. Urge the family to do the same. Try to make bargains or contracts with uncooperative patients, by dividing tasks into smaller parts. The patient with a hip replacement who's afraid to get out of bed, for instance, may agree to slide to the side and sit up. Whenever it's possible, offer him choices, such as whether he wants to try getting out of bed in the morning or in the afternoon.

When a patient is particularly difficult, schedule a conference to discuss the problem with the attending physician, nursing supervisor, any colleagues who also care for him, and, possibly, a social worker or psych nurse. In some hospitals, the RN who has the best relationship with the patient assumes primary care, in hopes that he'll benefit from having someone he knows he can count on.

Being nice to suit-prone patients and families isn't enough, though. You've got to carefully document every attempt you make to reach out to a troubled patient, and the results of each intervention as well. Don't gripe or gossip about that "horrible" patient. Avoid using derogatory labels in the nurses' notes. If any complication or injury occurs, such labels allow an attorney to argue that the patient received poor nursing care because the nurses didn't like him.

To chart behavior that's hostile, uncooperative, or uncommunicative, describe the patient's actions objectively. "turned her head away every time I talked to her," for instance, is more accurate than calling her hostile. "Refused to be repositioned throughout the shift" clearly indicates non-compliance. If the behavior carries a medical risk—the patient who refuses to be turned is at risk for pressure sores, for example—alert the doctor. Chart the call and note the physician's response.

There are times, however, when a good offense—being on the lookout for difficult patients, taking steps to defuse their anger, and careful documentation—may not be enough to forestall a suit. In this book we give you the tools you need to identify and avoid the legal danger spots in every area of your practice. Armed with this valuable information, you can continue to function effectively as a competent, caring nurse while protecting your license from suit-prone patients and their over-eager attorneys.

Medication errors: Learn from your colleagues' mistakes

A look at errors that have resulted in legal entanglements can help you avoid medication mistakes and the slew of consequences that may follow.

Roughly one out of every 100 doses of medication administered to hospital patients is done so in error, according to the American Society of Health-System Pharmacists. While no nurse is infallible herself, every nurse is in a position to intercept the errors of others— made during prescribing, transcribing, or dispensing. In fact, one study found that nurses are the ones most likely to catch medication errors, especially those made by physicians.[1]

Failing to detect a medication error, or making one yourself, has more repercussions than you might imagine. If the error results in injury, a malpractice claim leveled against you and your employer is a good bet. Among the other possibilities: disciplinary action, denial of unemployment benefits, an investigation of your facility's quality procedures by the state peer review organization, and payment issues related to treatment expenses.

Let's look at some actual medication errors to see how costly mistakes can be avoided.

Wrong substance

A patient in a Delaware hospital was scheduled to receive an injection of Lasix. When the nurse went to the stockroom to get the drug she mistakenly took a bottle of potassium chloride, instead.[2] After administering the medication, she noticed that the patient "looked funny." The patient arrested, resuscitation was unsuccessful, and the patient's estate sued for wrongful death.

In Colorado, a 2-year-old was given an adult dose of morphine, rather than a pediatric dose of codeine as per written orders.[3] The child was successfully resuscitated but suffered a speech defect and learning disabilities. The hospital agreed to an out-of-court settlement.

Errors like these can be prevented by reviewing the medication against the original order and reading the drug label carefully. If the order is unclear, incomplete, or hard to read, be sure to ask for clarification from the physician who wrote it.

If the order seems inappropriate, consult with the pharmacist, other nurses, or the literature. If you don't find the answers you're looking for, hold off on giving the medication until you've checked the order with the doctor who prescribed it.

Always double-check the name of the drug, especially if it looks or sounds similar to another one—like digoxin and digitoxin, or quinine and quinidine. Frequently, phenobarbital and pentobarbital are accidentally interchanged; not only do the names look and sound alike, but the indications are similar.

Access to drugs that are frequently associated with serious medication errors or have a narrow margin of safety should be restricted. Many hospitals store these drugs in an entirely different location. Potassium chloride, for example, may be available only in premixed IV containers through the pharmacy or from a nursing supervisor permitted to obtain it.

While floor-stock medications are convenient, they may set the stage for mistakes since there is no protective check by a pharmacist. Re-examine each one of the drugs stocked on the floor to see whether it is really medically necessary to have it so readily available.

Always review patients' charts for contraindications, such as a drug allergy. Listen to patients who question or object to a particular drug. If a patient says his pills are usually a different color, double-check the order and the medication dispensed by the pharmacy. Educating patients about prescribed medications is a key strategy for preventing errors.

Wrong dose

A nurse at an Illinois hospital injected a patient with 2 gm of lidocaine (Xylocaine), instead of the 100 mg that had been ordered.[4] She was found negligent, but one of the issues at trial was whether the packaging of the two different dosages in similar pre-filled syringes was confusing and contributed to the error.

An Ohio nurse administered a 30 mg IV dose of gentamicin (Garamycin, G-Mycin, Jenamicin) to a child, as prescribed.[5] Although the nurse thought the IV line was clamped when she left, the entire bottle—200 mg—of gentamicin infused over the next two hours. The nurse was found negligent for the child's hearing loss caused by the overdose.

In a Wisconsin case, a freeflow of lidocaine occurred when a hospital patient's IV line was not put back into an infusion pump after its removal. The patient died from the overdose, and the state peer review organization cited the hospital with a Level III quality concern, the most severe rating it could receive. Such citations can result in sanctions against the facility.

A patient in Alaska suffered a cardiac arrest after a nurse mistakenly administered an overdose of lidocaine.[6] At the direction of the attending physician, the patient's records were altered in an attempt to cover up the error; but another physician informed the patient's family about the overdose. They sued the attending physician and the hospital for malpractice and fraud.

Dosage errors can be avoided by double-checking all calculations, including dosage, flow rates, and anything else that requires the use of a mathematical formula. Make sure all decimal points are placed correctly, and never begin a notation with a decimal point because it can be easily overlooked; write 0.1 mg, for example, not .1 mg. If you are unsure of your results, have a colleague recheck the calculation.

Be sure to question unusual orders, particularly for large doses. If more than two tablets, capsules, ampuls, or other forms of a drug are required for one dose, chances are that too much medication is being prepared. Whenever a dosage is questionable, recheck the written order or check the dosage with the pharmacy. This is especially important with antineoplastic medications, since doses for these drugs are less standardized.

Read labels especially carefully if large amounts with several zeros are involved. If the dosage on the drug label is confusing, as in the Illinois case, alert the pharmacist so he can replace the label with one that is clearer. The pharmacy should also be encouraged to purchase a less error-prone product. If multidose vials are confusing, the pharmacy may be able to supply single-dose containers or add a cautionary label to the multidose vial.

Different drug dosages with similar packaging should not be stored next to one another. Keeping them apart will minimize the chances of someone grabbing the wrong concentration.

As a final precaution, be extra careful when using equipment such as multiple IV lines and infusion pumps. Routinely double-check each step of medication administration to assure that the equipment is functioning, manual administration sets are adjusted correctly, and lines are placed properly in pump devices.

Wrong route

A nurse at a Kansas hospital was found negligent for injecting Dramamine into the hip of an obese patient with a needle that was too short.[7] The patient developed a necrotic lesion because the medication was given subcutaneously rather than intramuscularly.

In Vermont, a nurse starting her shift noticed that a nurse on the previous shift had neglected to give a patient a dose of Decadron, as ordered. Thinking it was in the patient's best interest to administer the prescribed medication in the fastest way, she injected the drug IV push instead of administering by drip.[8]

Although the patient suffered no adverse effects, the nurse was terminated, and a state employment board denied her unemployment compensation benefits on the basis that she was guilty of misconduct. A court reversed that decision on appeal.

In Arkansas, a patient who was hospitalized for a work-related injury was given Maalox intravenously rather than orally by a student nurse. The patient's insurer refused to pay the hospital for any expenses related to the medication error. The state workers' compensation commission backed the insurer, finding that charges stemming from the error did not meet the payment standard of being "reasonable and necessary."[9]

Although the Arkansas case may sound unusual, patients have died after oral medications like Kaopectate, Metamucil, and Maalox were inserted into an IV line rather than a feeding tube.

Wrong route errors can be avoided by following established procedures for each route of administration, including using the right length needle. Use recommended landmarks for intramuscular injections. Always clarify any questionable routes with the physician.

Errors such as the one that occurred in Arkansas can be avoided if unnecessary IV lines are removed, and all necessary lines are clearly labeled. Trace each catheter from its insertion site to its most distal point, including the IV bag or bottle, before administering a drug. This can reduce the possibility that IV medication will be injected into an epidural catheter, or that oral medication will inadvertently be administered into a parenteral line.

Wrong time

An 86-year-old Texas patient was prescribed ibuprofen every four hours, but his nurse administered two doses within an hour and 15 minutes of each other.[10] The patient become unconscious as a result, and his stomach had to be pumped to revive him. The nurse was fired and denied unemployment benefits by the Texas Employment Commission because of his misconduct.

In Delaware, the state board of nursing found an LPN guilty of unprofessional conduct for double-medicating patients, falsely indicating in charts that medications had been given, and failing to document medications that had been given.[11] His license was suspended for three years.

In a Utah case, a nurse delayed a stat dose of the antipsychotic Mellaril for two hours.[12] Later that night, the patient jumped from the window of his room in an attempt to commit suicide and was permanently paralyzed.

Although timely administration of medications can be hampered by "system" problems such as insufficient nursing personnel or delayed transcription of orders, medication doses should be administered within 30 minutes of the time due. Speak to your supervisor if staffing problems are preventing you from doing this.

Don't hesitate to question an order if its timing seems inappropriate. Omit or delay a dose only when indicated by a specific condition or situation, and notify the physician promptly.

The five rights

A good foundation for preventing medication errors is observing the time-honored five "rights" taught in nursing school: Make sure you have the right patient (verify the patient's identity by checking his ID bracelet and asking him his name if possible), right drug, right dosage, right route, and right time.

In spite of—or maybe because of—the fact that these "rights" are so basic and simple, they are all too often overlooked. Following them religiously will prove invaluable in keeping errors to a minimum and avoiding legal pitfalls.

REFERENCES

1. Leape, L. L., Bates, D. W., et al. (1995). Systems Analysis of Adverse Drug Events, JAMA, 274(1), 35.
2. Ciarlo v. St. Francis Hospital, 1994 WL 713864 (Del. Super).
3. Neves v. Potters 769 P.2d 1047 (1989).
4. Wingstrom v. Evanston Hospital, 1992 WL 97934 (N.D. Ill.).
5. Gallimore v. Children's Hospital Medical Center, 1992 WL 37742 (Ohio App. 1 Dist.).
6. Sharrow v. Archer, 658 P.2d 1331 (1983).
7. Barnes v. St. Francis Hospital, 211 Kan. 315, 507 P.2d 288 (1973).
8. Porter v. Department of Employment Security, 139 Vt. 405, 430 A.2d 450 (1981).
9. Tracor v. Baptist Medical Center, 29 Ark. App. 198, 780 WS.W.2d 26 (1989).
10. Hagger v. The Texas Employment Commission, 1995 WL 82050 (Tex. App. Hous. 1 Dist.).
11. Hicks v. State of Delaware, 1994 WL 164507 (1994).
12. Farrow v. Health Services, et al, 604 P.2d 474 (1979).

When IV practice spells *mal* practice

IV therapy presents liability risks for nurses both in and out of the hospital. You'll want to avoid the mistakes that could come back to haunt you.

More and more nurses are finding themselves on the witness stand in IV-related malpractice cases. That's not surprising given some recent trends: Intravenous equipment and therapies have become more complex, many IV teams have been disbanded, and the ranks of those receiving IV therapy have swelled to eight patients in 10.[1]

What lands nurses in legal hot water most often—and the focus of this article—is infiltration and extravasation. Extravasation is the inadvertent administration of a vesicant solution—like dopamine or many chemotherapeutic agents, which cause blisters, necrosis, and sloughing—into the surrounding tissue instead of the vein. Infiltration is the inadvertent administration of a nonvesicant solution into the surrounding tissue.

Other complications that provoke lawsuits include phlebitis, air embolism, breakage of peripherally inserted central catheters (PICCs), and hematomas that cause nerve compression injuries.

If you care for patients receiving IV therapy—in a hospital, clinic, doctor's office, or the home—you need to know what the liability risks are, and how to defend yourself if something does go wrong.

Preventing molehills from becoming mountains

The occurrence of either infiltration or extravasation doesn't in and of itself amount to negligence. That determination hinges on how much solution has entered the tissue, how quickly you detected the problem, and what you did to correct it.

If, for example, you observe swelling right after a solution begins infusing, and you stop the infusion immediately and remove the vascular access device, you'd be acting as a prudent nurse should.

On the other hand, if the first sign of trouble you see is 2+ pitting edema from the patient's wrist to the forearm, a plaintiff's attorney can make a strong case for nursing negligence if injury results. Accumulation of a large amount of fluid over a long period of time—and there are equations that attorneys will use to determine exactly how long—suggests that neither the patient nor the infusion were being monitored properly.

With vesicants, escape of even a small amount of fluid into surrounding tissue can be harmful, and the damage permanent. Damage from nonvesicants—which can also be permanent—often depends on how much has infiltrated. A large amount can cause nerve compression, resulting in numbness or paralysis in an extremity. In addition, a fasciotomy may be needed to relieve fluid pressure in the tissue. The surgery will result in scarring.

To prevent injury, inspect the IV site regularly in accordance with your employer's policy, and routinely ask the patient how the IV site feels. While swelling is the hallmark of infiltration and extravasation, pain or discomfort around the vascular access device is also common. The accumulation of fluid may also produce numbness and tingling in the arm, often radiating down to the fingers.

Be sure to troubleshoot all patient reports of pain or discomfort. They may also signal one of the other IV-related complications that trigger lawsuits. Pain around the cannula, for instance, is usually a precursor of phlebitis.[2]

Air embolism, another preventable IV-related complication, can result from failing to properly occlude the insertion site after removing a central line. In one case involving a hospital in Pennsylvania, an RN removed a patient's central line at her supervisor's request—then simply applied a gauze pressure dressing.

The patient fell out of bed as he was being turned, and then quickly coded: Air had been sucked into his circulatory system through the gauze, causing a stroke that proved fatal. The hospital ultimately paid a $3 million settlement.

Are your practices up to snuff?

Regardless of which IV-related complication triggers a lawsuit, the jury will be trying to determine one thing if you are sued— whether you upheld the standard of care.

If you are the one who inserted the vascular access device, be prepared to explain the clinical criteria you used for choosing the insertion site. Answers like, "I couldn't find any other vein," or "That's the vein I always use," won't hold up in court.

According to the standards of the Intravenous Nurses Society (INS)—and you will be expected to know them—vein selection should be based on an assessment of the patient's condition, age, and diagnosis; vein condition, size, and location; and the type and duration of therapy.[2]

You will also be expected to know the venous anatomy and physiology of the hand, arm, and chest, and to name the vein you accessed—cephalic, basilic, or median antebrachial, for example. Be prepared to justify the type and gauge of device you selected, as well.

If you were responsible for monitoring the infusion, you will have to explain how you determined that the vascular access device was working properly. Any nurse caring for a patient receiving IV therapy must be able to recognize and troubleshoot equipment problems. That ability is especially important with infusion pumps, since most pumps continue to infuse solution even after the surrounding tissue becomes filled with fluid.

If you're asked to work with an electronic infusion device that you are not familiar with, request training from your employer or the manufacturer of the device.

You must also be familiar with the type of medication being infused, including possible side effects and specific interventions. Some solutions are, in and of themselves, harmless if they enter the tissue; others require an antidote to prevent damage such as tissue sloughing. In an Oklahoma case involving dopamine extravasation, the hospital had to pay millions of dol-

lars in damages because the nurses did not know the antidote—
phentolamine (Regitine)—or that it had to be administered
within 12 hours of the extravasation.[3]

In addition to knowing the INS standards, make sure that you
are familiar with and follow the IV therapy policies and procedures of your employer. If those policies do not reflect the standards of nursing practice, request an update.

Document your request—to whom you made it and when—in
a memo to yourself. This memo could prove valuable if a problem
arises because you weren't supplied with an appropriate policy
statement.

Your documentation: Concise is better

Whenever you start an IV, document the date and time that you
did so and name the vein that you accessed. In one malpractice
case, the nurse had just charted "upper left arm," leaving doubts
about which vein had been accessed—and her abilities.

Also chart the gauge, length, style, and brand of the needle
or catheter, and whether the solution was being delivered by
gravity infusion or a pump. Note the rate of flow.

Document each insertion attempt. A record of repeated
unsuccessful attempts can indicate that the patient has poor
peripheral vein access.

Use the patient's own comments about discomfort—or lack of
it—in your charting. Words like "my arm feels fine" will provide
a much stronger defense than your opinion that "the patient tolerated the procedure well."

Chart each one of your assessments. Describe all of the signs
and symptoms in detail. If an infiltration occurs, for example,
estimate the amount of fluid that entered the tissues if at all possible. If you are not sure, measure the area of infiltration.

Document the location of the infiltration, too, either in
words—"swollen from fingers to antecubital fossa"—or by drawing the limb and shading the affected area. Take care to be
accurate, though.

Chart all actions you took in response to indications of a problem, including notification of the physician. Whenever you remove a device, document why.

Watchwords: Education and preparedness

Home care nurses need to do more than nurse their patients who are on IV therapy; they also need to be risk managers. Education of the patient and his family is paramount.

Make sure they know the signs and symptoms of possible complications, the appropriate interventions, and emergency procedures. Be certain they know how to contact health care personnel 24 hours a day. Reevaluate their knowledge on a periodic basis.

Reinforce your teaching by giving the patient written reference material; attorneys in IV-related home care malpractice cases often request this information. If your home care agency does not provide written instructions—and many do not—request that it do so.

Document your teaching, ideally by using a checklist form that both you and the patient sign. Also document your assessment of the level of understanding exhibited by the patient and his family members. If you think a patient's abilities or level of comprehension disqualifies him as a candidate for home infusion therapy, document this judgment and notify your supervisor.

Make certain that you know how to contact your supervisor at all times, and—in case it ever becomes necessary—how to move a concern upwards through the chain of command. Keep a copy of your employer's policy and procedure manual with you.

Also be mindful of clinical strategies that may be inappropriate. For example, administering a vesicant solution through a peripheral line may be an option for hospitalized patients who have pumps. But, for patients at home, the high risk of extravasation and the lack of continuous nursing supervision make a central line the safest choice in this situation.

Although there are no definitive guidelines on the need for home care nurses to get informed consent,[4] I'd advise any home care nurse who's accessing the venous system to obtain it. This is the general practice among nurses who perform PICC insertions, and is increasingly becoming so among those who do routine peripheral IV insertion site rotations.

The legal risks associated with IV therapy can be high. But concise documentation, thorough patient teaching, and a working knowledge of the standards of care can knock those risks down considerably.

REFERENCES

1. Masoorli, S. (1995). Infusion therapy lawsuits: An occupational hazard. Journal of Intravenous Nursing, 18(2), 88.
2. Intravenous Nurses Society. (1990). Intravenous nursing standards of practice. Belmont, MA: Author.
3. Malseed, R., & Harrigan G. (1989). Textbook of pharmacology and nursing care, Philadelphia: J. B. Lippincott, 239-240.
4. Sullivan, G. H. (1994). Home Care: More autonomy, more legal risks. RN, 57(5), 63.

If equipment causes injury

Manufacturers, hospitals, and nurses all play a role in preventing equipment-related injuries. Knowing what your duties are will help protect both you and your patient.

A 5-month-old boy begins shivering in the recovery room after routine surgery. A nurse places the baby on a heating pad to warm him. During a diaper change later that day, the nurse discovers large blisters on the baby's buttocks. A physician diagnoses second- and third-degree burns.[1]

A patient's oxygen supply is unplugged from the wall outlet so she can be transferred to a private room nearby. Nurses attempt to connect the oxygen supply to the outlet in the patient's new room, but a permanent light fixture next to the outlet makes insertion of the oxygen flow meter impossible. As the nurses rush to find a portable oxygen unit, the patient goes into respiratory arrest and dies minutes later.[2]

A day after a patient undergoes open-heart surgery a nurse notices that his chest dressing is wet, and notifies the physician. An examination reveals serious chemical burns to the patient's chest and abdominal walls, the result of nitroprusside (Nipride) leaking through a hole in the atrial catheter during surgery.[3]

Any medical device—whether it's as simple as a heating pad, as familiar as a catheter, or as complex as a ventilator—can be dangerous if it malfunctions or is used incorrectly. Not having the right equipment available when it's needed can be just as costly.

According to Food and Drug Administration officials, the FDA received 112,000 reports of serious illness, injury, or death involving medical devices over a recent 12-month period. About a third of those reports stemmed from the use of breast implants.

Who is legally at fault when a medical device harms instead of helps: The manufacturer? The health care facility? The physician? Or the nurse? And what precautions should you take to prevent injury and liability in the first place?

Where the law assigns responsibility

The burns the baby suffered from the heating pad were not caused by any product defect. The pad was not designed for infants, and even carried a warning label stating so. The nurse's negligence in using the pad was the sole cause of the injury, and the hospital agreed to pay a settlement to the child's parents.

Even if the heating pad had been designed for infants and a defect in the product had resulted in the burns, the nurse could still have been held liable if she had failed to inspect the product before use to detect any obvious defects—such as a frayed cord—or if she had spotted or suspected a defect but used the product anyway.

Manufacturers, like nurses, face liability if they knew or should have known that a product was defective or unsafe. Any manufacturer who knows about a safety problem has a duty to notify users or, if appropriate, remove the product from the market.

Take, for example, the case of the patient who suffered intra-operative chemical burns. He sued three of his surgeons and the manufacturer of the catheter. The jury found that the hole in the catheter was not the result of negligence by the doctors. Instead, it held the manufacturer liable for failing to warn surgeons that the catheter could be punctured if the tube was threaded backwards—through the needle point to the hub—as had been done in this case.

One of the issues disputed at trial was whether the manufacturer had an obligation to warn users about this particular danger or whether the surgeons should have known about it without being told. Courts have held that manufacturers have no duty to warn users about obvious hazards—such as the risk of sustaining a needlestick from recapping a needle.

Health care facilities, too, have a duty to warn: They must inform staff about any safety alerts received from manufacturers or regulatory agencies such as the FDA. In one case, for example, a hospital failed to notify nurses of a manufacturer's alert that the automatic lowering device on electric beds for pediatric patients needed to be disabled. When a child was crushed to death after activating the device, the liability fell entirely on the hospital's shoulders.

Health care facilities are also responsible for having all necessary equipment on hand and ensuring that it's in working order. In the instance of the woman who died when her oxygen supply couldn't be hooked up—a notable equipment liability case—the hospital was found at fault. The court ruled that the facility's negligence in having neither a working oxygen supply in the new room nor a portable oxygen unit available during the patient's transfer led to her death.

Taking precautions to ensure patients' safety

Since nurses are responsible for using equipment correctly and preventing defective equipment from being used, certain safety measures are a necessary part of your routine.

Carefully inspect all equipment before use. If you spot a defect, report it right away to your unit manager and the engineering or biomedical department. Affix a "do not use" sticker to the device and a note stating what's wrong with it. Fill out an incident report detailing the problem.

You are not usually responsible for detecting equipment defects that aren't obvious; however there could be times when you are. Here's an example: A leak in the balloon of an indwelling catheter allowed urine to contaminate a patient's skin graft, necessitating additional surgeries. A jury found an OR nurse negligent because she did not test the balloon for holes before the catheter was inserted.[4]

With that in mind, make sure you are familiar with manufacturer recommendations and current nursing practice on equipment checks, and act accordingly. Read and follow all cautionary labels on equipment. Never modify a device or use it for anything other than its intended purpose.

Unless an emergency compels you to do so, refrain from using equipment that you lack the skill and knowledge to operate. Insist on thorough training.

Investigate the possibility of a malfunction or user error if readings from equipment, such as an EKG or a blood glucose monitor, do not jibe with the patient's overall clinical picture. Try switching to another device or recalibrating the machine. If you still suspect the device is not working properly, stop using it, tag it, and notify the appropriate personnel.

When medical equipment is used in the home

With more and more sophisticated devices being used in home care, educating patients and their families about the proper use and maintenance of equipment is especially important. Provide verbal and hands-on instruction, and supplement it with written material. Ask for return demonstrations. Make sure patients know how to correct equipment problems and who to contact if they're unable to. Document all of your teaching.

It helps if patients receive reference material about the particular device they are using. Unfortunately, many manufacturers' instruction manuals are too complex and technical for lay users. You may want to develop your own user manual to give out to patients, although doing so creates a liability risk if you don't communicate the manufacturer's instructions accurately or completely.[5]

To minimize the potential for liability, have your facility's risk manager and the manufacturer's representative review any instructions you write, and document that you have done so. In addition, consider how understandable a manufacturer's user manual is when recommending brands to your patients for purchase.

How to respond to problems

Whenever equipment misuse or malfunction results in injury, taking care of the patient is, of course, your top priority. Once you have done that, notify the patient's doctor, your supervisor, and your facility's biomedical or engineering department.

Retain the equipment and any broken parts so they can be examined later. Document all your actions and complete an incident report.

If an equipment problem caused or contributed to a death or serious illness or injury, the Safe Medical Devices Act (SMDA) requires that the health care facility report the incident to the FDA and, in some cases, to the manufacturer. This law does not apply to physicians' offices.

If you work in a doctor's office, or if you work for a health care facility and have any safety concerns about a device that do not require mandatory reporting under the SMDA, consider making a report to MedWatch, the FDA's voluntary program for reporting adverse events related to medical devices and drugs.

According to FDA officials, Medwatch has received some 5,900 reports of problems with medical devices since it began in 1993—20% of them have come from nurses. For more information, call the MedWatch hotline, (800) FDA-1088.

What if you're the one who's hurt

Given the array of devices nurses handle, equipment-related injuries can be considered an occupational hazard. If you are hurt as a result of faulty equipment, you have the right to sue the manufacturer, just as patients do. If a separate company serviced the product and poor repair or maintenance was to blame, you can sue that company.

Whether the injury was the result of malfunction or misuse—even on your part—you are eligible for workers' compensation. However, if you are covered by workers' comp, the law precludes you from suing your employer even if negligence on your employer's part caused the injury.

Hopefully, you won't ever have a reason to think about suing. By using equipment correctly and taking all the necessary precautions, you can minimize the likelihood of injury for you, your colleagues, and your patients.

REFERENCES

1. Beckmann, J. P. (1995). Problems associated with equipment and products. In Nursing malpractice (pp. 186-193). Seattle: University of Washington Press.
2. Bellaire General Hospital v. Campbell, 510 S.W. 2nd 94 (TX, 1974).
3. Knowlton v. Deseret Med., Inc., 930 F.2d 116 (1991, U.S. App.).
4. Richard v. Southwest Louisiana Hospital Association, 383 So. 2d 83 (La. Ct. App. 1980).
5. Kingsley, P. A., Backinger, C. K., & Brady, M. W. (1995). Medical-device user instructions. Home Healthcare Nurse, 13(1), 31.

Restraints:
A legal catch-22?

They can protect patients, or injure them.
You could be sued for using them, or for failing to.

Nurses use restraints to protect patients from falling, wandering, or pulling out invasive devices. Yet they are the cause of an estimated 200 deaths and many more injuries each year, generally in elderly patients.[1] In some instances, a restraint should not have been used in the first place. In others, misuse—selecting the wrong restraint, applying it incorrectly, or keeping it on too long—is to blame.

To safeguard patients in long-term care facilities, the federal government, as part of the 1987 Omnibus Budget Reconciliation Act (OBRA), regulated the use of restraints including arm and leg restraints, hand mitts, soft ties or safety vests, wheelchair safety bars, and geri-chairs.[2]

Then the FDA jumped on the bandwagon, prompted by increasing numbers of reports of fractures, burns, and deaths from asphyxiation. In November 1991, the agency issued a warning on restraints and a long list of recommendations, which apply to acute care as well as long-term care.

One recommendation calls for every institution to have—and communicate—protocols for the use of restraints. If your facility doesn't have such a policy or you're not familiar with it, discuss the problem with your supervisor or risk manager.

Try these alternatives before you restrain

The safety of your patient or others should be the only reason to consider a protective device. Although it's often easier and quicker to apply restraints than to try alternatives, OBRA states clearly that they should be a last resort, not applied for the convenience of the staff.

Some alternatives are not very time consuming at all. Try wedging pads of pillows against the sides of a wheelchair to keep a patient properly positioned, for example. A removable lap tray may provide support, and keep some patients in place as well.

If a patient becomes disoriented as darkness falls—a phenomenon known as sundown syndrome—look for physical problems such as poor hearing or eyesight that might contribute to his confusion. Try soft music, a warm beverage, soft lights, or a back rub to quiet agitated patients. Spend some extra time with a restless patient, or ask a family member to stay by his side until he falls asleep.

Some nursing homes have begun to use what are called "environmental" restraints. Large plants or pieces of furniture act as barriers to prevent patients from wandering beyond designated areas. A picture or personal possession hung on the door to a patient's room, for instance, can prevent him from getting lost. Positioning beds closer to the floor makes falling out less dangerous.

When more protection is needed, OBRA requires that restraints be applied only under a doctor's written order, one that specifies why the restraint is needed and for how long it will be used. The FDA makes a similar recommendation.

Communicate with doctor, family, and patient

Despite these guidelines, a recent study shows that 75% of the time nurses are the ones who decide when to apply restraints.[3] Often, they have standing orders that allow the use of restraints under certain circumstances, provided they get a written order from the physician within 24 hours. The study showed, however, that in many cases, attending physicians were never told that their patients had been restrained. If your institution has such a policy, be sure to comply, for safety reasons and your own legal protection.

Federal regulations also require that patients agree to be restrained. In seeking consent, explain the reason for the restraint. Point out that you've tried other alternatives. If the patient is incompetent, talk to his family members or healthcare proxy. If patient or proxy refuses the device despite a detailed explanation of why it's needed, document the conversation, and report the problem to your supervisor at once.

During a life-threatening emergency, of course, you can restrain a patient without his permission. Similarly, no special permission is needed to restrain him during a treatment he's already consented to. In either case, remove the restraint as soon as you've completed the treatment.

Caregivers should begin planning for the removal of a restraint as soon as it's applied. While restraints are in place, monitor patients carefully. Remove the restraint and exercise and reposition the patient at least every two hours. Prolonged immobility has been associated with a host of conditions, including dehydration, pressure sores, depression, nosocomial infection, and incontinence.[3,4]

Select the type of restraint with caution

Nurses not only make the decision about when to restrain patients, but choose the restraint to apply. The rule of thumb here: Use the least restrictive device that will keep the patient safe. Using a vest, for instance, when a soft wrist restraint would be sufficient to prevent a frail, elderly patient from wandering increases the possibility that he will fall or become entangled in the device.

No matter what kind of restraint you're considering, keep in mind that whether you use a restraint or fail to use use one, there is a potential legal risk.

In one case, for instance, a patient in a safety vest tumbled out of bed and broke her hip, then sued the hospital for the actions of the nurse who restrained her.[5] On the other hand, another patient, injured when she fell our of her wheelchair, successfully sued the facility because staff members failed to provide a restraining device.[6]

To help prevent injury and liability, the FDA urges caregivers to post instructions for the use of restraints in a prominent location, and follow directions to the letter. Among other recommendations:

- Select the appropriate device for the patient's condition.
- Check weight and height requirements to be sure the device is the right size.
- Check the positioning of the restraint, particularly the front and back.
- Tie knots that release easily to ensure quick access.
- Secure bed restraints to the bed springs or frame, not to the mattress or side rails. If the bed is adjustable, prevent constriction by securing the restraints to the parts of the bed that move with the patient.[7]

Document interventions and outcomes

Documentation, always important, is essential in situations in which restraints are involved. Record each attempt to safeguard or calm the patient without restraining him, as well as each outcome. If a patient requires a restraint because his condition has deteriorated, document the decline. The record should demonstrate that you followed your facility's policies and procedures.

In long-term care, surveyors from government agencies will look for evidence that use of the restraint has been limited to brief periods of time for specific purposes—or that the patient's physical and mental condition hasn't deteriorated since he's been restrained.

If a patient has been restrained for more than two hours at a time, chart each time he's released, taken to the toilet, and monitored for skin breakdown.

In short, your documentation should reflect your guiding principle when considering and applying restraints: These protective devices are the exception, not the rule.

REFERENCES

1. Staff. (1991, September). Alert targets geriatric restraints. ATLA Advocate, (17)6, 1.

2. Staff. (1990). OBRA and physical restraints: What the regulations mean.

3. Macpherson, D.S., Lofgren, R.P., et al. (1990). Deciding to restrain medical patients. J. AM. Geriatr. Soc., (38)5, 516.

4. Ramsay, W.A. (1990, April 1). Use of restraints opposed in nursing homes. The Sunday Star-Ledger, Health/Fitness, 11.

5. Keys v. Tallahassee Memorial Regional Medical Center, 579 S. 2d 201 (FL 1991).

6. Kujawski v. Arbor View Health Care Center, 407 N.W. 2d 249 (WI 1987).

7. Food and Drug Administration. (1991, November 14). Potential hazards with protective restraint devices. (MDA91-3). Rockville, MD: FDA Medical Alert.

When language is an obstacle

The variety of languages spoken by health care providers and patients alike raises a myriad of legal questions. Neither the issues—nor the answers—are clearcut.

Working in an ethnically diverse setting is an enriching experience. But if a language barrier prevents you from understanding a co-worker or patient—or keeps someone from understanding you—your patient's safety could be at stake.

Whether and when an individual may be required to speak English is a sensitive and controversial issue that's bound to raise questions: If English is your second language, for instance, do you have the right to converse with your colleagues in your native tongue? If a health care provider you're working with has limited English skills, are you obligated to intervene? How far must you go to accommodate patients or their family members who don't speak English?

The law isn't always clear on these issues and it by no means affords blanket protection to employees who speak a foreign language on the job—or even those who speak English with a heavy accent. Several important court cases reveal just how murky aspects of the language issue really are.

Knowing what your professional duty demands and the legal basis for it will help you safeguard patients, lessen your risk of liability, and increase your job security.

The validity of English-only rules

Suppose several nurses on your unit frequently converse in their native language at the nurses station, in the lounge, and in front of patients. This has produced tension among staff and complaints from patients. Can your supervisor require all employees to speak English at all times?

Probably not. Strict English-only rules in the workplace that prohibit workers from speaking a foreign language even while on breaks or at lunch are likely to violate Title VII of the Civil Rights Act of 1965, which prohibits employment discrimination based on national origin.

The Equal Employment Opportunity Commission (EEOC), the agency that administers Title VII, maintains that an individual's primary language is an essential characteristic of national origin. So, courts may view English-only policies as harassment, a burdensome condition of employment, or discriminatory.

However, EEOC guidelines may permit policies that require employees to speak English while they are on duty—provided the employer can show that such a policy is a business necessity compelling enough to override any racial impact. Legitimate business needs that courts have recognized include promoting employee efficiency, productivity, and safety; maintaining order and discipline; and responding to customer preference.

The case of an assistant head nurse in California who filed a Title VII action against her employer is one example: The hospital had prohibited the nurse and those she supervised from speaking their native Filipino dialect of Tagalog on the maternity unit where they worked.

The rule was necessary, hospital administrators asserted, because conversations in Tagalog had resulted in preferential treatment for the nurses who spoke it and adversely affected worker morale and supervision. The court found that the language restriction did not violate the nurse's civil rights because it was motivated by a desire to eliminate dissension that could have compromised patient safety.[1]

Foreign accents and patient safety

Let's say you're working with a doctor who has a heavy accent. You have a tough time making out his verbal orders, and he gets angry when you ask him to repeat himself. Patient safety is definitely at issue if communication is hampered by the doctor's accent.

Despite Title VII employee protection, there are instances where an accent may be a legitimate basis for job actions, including firing or refusing to hire someone. In one hotly debated case, a court in Hawaii upheld a decision by Honolulu's motor vehicle department not to hire a clerk because he had a heavy accent: The recruiters believed the applicant's accent would have hampered his ability to communicate with the public—an essential requirement of the job.[2]

While people with thick accents may have a tough time getting hired, the threat of legal action deters most employers from dismissing an employee on that basis. In the case of an attending physician who is not a hospital employee, termination isn't even an option.

Fortunately, there are usually less drastic alternatives. In the case of telephone orders, technology may help. Many nursing units and doctors' offices are equipped with fax machines or are linked by computer networks. The doctor with the accent can be asked to enter the order on the computer or to fax it.

If a fax or computer order isn't an option, confirm the doctor's order by repeating it back to him. Do the same thing with in-person verbal orders. Either way, write the order in the chart and ask for the doctor's signature as soon as possible, or follow your hospital's policy for telephone and in-person verbal orders.

Whatever the situation, you must be firm in requiring that the physician provide comprehensible information. A doctor has a legal duty to give clear, intelligible verbal and written orders. However, heavy accents—or doctors' notoriously poor penmanship, for that matter—do not excuse you from your duty to clarify a poorly communicated order.

Your role as patient advocate is also central here. If you believe a patient is being denied the information he needs to make informed decisions because his doctor cannot communicate effectively, you may have an ethical duty to take action. If you are unsure, discuss the matter with your supervisor, a member of the ethics committee, or a patient care representative.

If you do decide to step in, objectively document the facts of the case and discuss the complaint with your supervisor. If she does not think the matter should be pursued but you still do, forward your complaint to the appropriate department—risk management or quality assessment, for example—or to the medical staff committee.

Keep in mind that nurses should not assume responsibility for providing patients with information necessary for informed consent. That is a legal duty which, with few exceptions, rests with the doctor.

What if the patient doesn't understand?

A patient who speaks broken English arrives at your outpatient facility shortly after fainting. You ask him whether he's on any medication and he shakes his head No. The doctor writes a prescription and the patient later experiences side effects caused by a drug interaction. It turns out the patient had been taking antibiotics but had not understood your question.

The Americans with Disabilities Act (ADA) and the Rehabilitation Act mandate that federally funded hospitals and other public facilities accommodate people who are deaf by finding ways to communicate with them. But the inability to speak or understand English is not considered a disability, and there is no comparable federal law requiring that accommodations be made for such patients.

Some states do have laws that require hospitals to provide interpreters for foreign-speaking patients.[3] But whether you work in one of those states or not, you are still obligated to meet the standard of care. JCAHO standards for ensuring patient rights include meeting their "communication needs."[4] The American Hospital Association's patient's bill of rights also states that hospitals must be sensitive to linguistic differences.[5]

That means you must make a reasonable effort to overcome language barriers. If you do not and the patient does not get the care he needs as a result, you are jeopardizing his safety and leaving yourself open to a negligence suit.

If you encounter a language problem, find out if a family member can translate or help communicate. Because you will be discussing personal medical information, ask the patient for his consent before using any interpreter, family member or not. Document the interpreter's name and relationship to the patient, if any.

When you provide patient education or discharge instructions, ask the patient to repeat what you have said to ensure you are understood. Back up your teaching with written instructions, too, preferably in the language the patient speaks, if possible.

Hospitals should have established procedures for communicating with their non-English speaking patients, such as maintaining and using a roster of employees who are willing to serve as interpreters or working with an outside interpreting service. The policy should also address confidentiality issues and the third party's lack of medical knowledge.

If your hospital doesn't have such a policy, talk to your supervisor or risk manager about developing one. If you care for a large number of foreign-born patients who speak a particular language, such as Spanish, consider taking an intensive language course. Besides finding it easier to communicate with patients, you may discover that learning about another culture has its own rewards.

REFERENCES

1. Dimaranan v. Pomona Valley Medical Center, et al., 775 F. Supp. 338 (C. D. Cal. 1991).
2. Fragante v. City and County of Honolulu, et al., 888 F.2d 591 (9th Cir. 1989).
3. Woloshin, S., Bickell, N. A., et al. (1995). Language barriers in medicine in the United States. JAMA, 273(9), 724.
4. The Joint Commission. (1994). 1995 Accreditation manual for hospitals: Vol. 1. Standards. Oakbrook Terrace, IL: Joint Commission on Accreditation of Healthcare Organizations.
5. American Hospital Association. (1992). A patient's bill of rights. Chicago: Author.

The legal perils of patient discharge

Cutting corners on a patient discharge—
no matter what a managed care company says—
could land you in a court of law.
Here's what you can do to prevent liability.

One evening some years ago a patient we'll call Mrs. Getz, an elderly woman with a history of epilepsy, arrived by ambulance at a crowded inner city ED. She thought that she was having a seizure, but her blood tests showed therapeutic levels of Dilantin, and the doctor who examined her decided she was well enough to go home.

But while she was waiting for the results of her blood work, Mrs. Getz had been wheeled off to a quiet corner of the ED. She sat there alone—unaware that the staff had complied with neither of her two requests to call her son—and virtually unnoticed. At 3 a.m., a half hour after the ED staff had officially discharged her, she had a mild seizure and slid off the wheelchair. She was helped off the floor by a passing aide and indicated that her son was coming soon, not realizing that he'd never been called. The aide wheeled her out to the deserted hospital lobby.

Mrs. Getz remained there, half asleep and still dazed, for three hours. Then, two security guards, most likely thinking that she was a homeless person because of her disheveled appearance, forcibly escorted her to a taxi-stand bench in front of the hospital.

There, she had another seizure, falling to the ground and sustaining cuts and bruises. Two good Samaritans brought her back into the emergency room, where she was readmitted to the ED—this time by the day staff.

Unfortunately, attorneys hear bizarre tales like this routinely. And they lead to successful malpractice suits. This case certainly did: The jury quickly returned a verdict of negligence against the ED nursing staff, ordering the hospital to pay $40,000 in damages. If Mrs. Getz's injuries had been severe, the award would have been considerably higher.

As managed care pressures to reduce lengths of stay build and staff cutbacks continue, the risk of a careless or inappropriate discharge—from the ED or any other unit—is higher than ever. Since nurses are smack in the middle of the liability chain, you need to know how to protect yourself and your patients.

Guarding against a premature discharge

Determining if a patient is medically ready to be discharged is the physician's responsibility. But assessing the patient's condition at discharge to make sure that she is well enough to leave is a duty that falls squarely on the nurse's shoulders. Failing to perform this evaluation—a glaring omission in Mrs. Getz's case—is one of the most common reasons nurses are found liable for negligent discharge.

Even a basic physical assessment would have revealed that Mrs. Getz couldn't walk on her own and had signs of a seizure—findings that should have been reported to the physician. In certain circumstances, a nurse's duty goes beyond just notifying the doctor of significant findings: Courts have ruled that the nurse must try to prevent a discharge she believes does not meet the standard of care.[1]

How do you make that determination? There is no sure-fire rule, but the forseeability and imminence of harm to the patient are key factors.

Consider the following case: Mr. Smith, also a pseudonym, saw his surgeon a few days after being sent home from the hospital in a cast, and complained that his toe was numb and cool. The doctor told him to "stop worrying so much." A few days later, Mr. Smith's necrotic toe was amputated.

Because the nursing staff had noted the toe pallor and coolness at discharge and had informed the surgeon, the physician was in legal hot water all by himself. But if Mr. Smith had had more ominous signs—a bluish color, for instance—and his nurses had not attempted to stop the discharge, they, too, would likely have been charged with negligence.

If you feel a condition is serious enough to preclude discharge, you must notify the physician. If she disagrees with your recommendation, report the situation to your supervisor. If your supervisor disagrees with you, too, and you still believe that it is unsafe to discharge the patient, take your concerns further up the chain of command. Document your notifications in the chart.

In cases like Mr. Smith's, where the danger is less certain and there is a post-hospitalization visit scheduled within a few days of discharge, you may be correct in deferring to the physician. But when in doubt, refer the matter to your supervisor.

The best protection rests with the chart

Even if Mrs. Getz's nurses had met the standard of care, there was no way to prove it; her chart contained no notes about the ongoing assessment that she should have received or her condition at discharge. Mr. Smith's nurses, on the other hand, had carefully charted his symptoms and the fact that they had alerted the surgeon.

Your nursing discharge notes should provide a written picture of the patient that will be as vivid and complete as a photograph shown to the jury. Review all body systems. Quote the patient when it's appropriate: "I'm feeling great. I haven't had any chest pain in days." This type of entry can be a valuable aid if the patient has a myocardial infarction a week later and the family sues for premature discharge.

To prove that your care met professional standards, also chart all abnormal signs, symptoms, and diagnostic results present the day before and the day of discharge. Document, too, which physician has been notified of them or personally observed them. Depending on hospital policy and the patient's acuity, the physician may have visited the patient as long as 20 hours before discharge, so record all doctors' visits on the day of discharge. Contact the physician if you feel he needs to see the patient before discharge.

Conversely, note all improvements in the patient's condition, normal vital signs, and the lack of any complications that could be reasonably anticipated, such as tissue discoloration in a limb with a newly applied cast. Note the exact time of discharge, which staff member was in attendance, and, if appropriate, who was going to care for the patient at home and any discharge referrals.

Identify and address discharge needs

Just as he is responsible for all the patient's care, the physician is responsible for determining how the patient's care will be managed after discharge, but the physician and nurse share responsibility for coordinating any necessary referrals. If you become aware of a potential problem with the patient's post-hospitalization care, you must resolve it or advise the physician. No amount of explanation will convince a jury if a simple conversation with the doctor could have avoided a life-long disability.

When you alert the doctor to the patient's discharge needs, document that you did so. If a representative of social service, home care, or other area is scheduled to show up and doesn't, follow up with them and document these efforts as well. If the patient's home care needs are acute, consider delaying the discharge until all the necessary resources are in place.

Nurses are responsible for making sure the patient and appropriate family members receive and understand discharge instructions, so don't neglect your role as educator even if pressed for time.

To avoid claims that the patient or family was not informed of key information, such as signs and symptoms to watch for, document all patient and family teaching and the discharge instructions you provide. Many ED protocols require patients to sign two-part carbonless forms that list important follow-up information; the patient takes one copy with him and the other is placed in the chart.

Finally, ask the patient how she will be getting home and then see that the appropriate person is called if necessary—an omission by Mrs. Getz's nurses that certainly didn't impress the jury. If there's a logistical problem, contact the social services department or follow your hospital's policy. Many facilities provide cab fare for patients who need it; some rural hospitals call local police to take patients home.

Making sure you perform in accord with the standards of your facility and national guidelines is the best way to protect yourself from liability—but it's not enough. How well you documented your actions can determine whether you receive a hearty nod of approval from the jury or a costly verdict against you.

REFERENCES

1. Fiesta, J. (1994). Premature discharge. Nursing Management, 25(4), 17.

When a patient refuses treatment

If a patient declines medical care, you need to take action—to protect the patient's health and insulate yourself from legal repercussions.

As nurses, we know that patients have the right to refuse treatment and leave the hospital at any time—that's what patient autonomy is all about. But what if the patient doesn't know or fully understand the consequences of his actions; what's a nurse's duty then? What if he's intoxicated, or suicidal; are you obligated to comply with his wishes? How about if he's a minor?

Because there isn't necessarily a single answer to questions like these, a review of the rules, the exceptions, and the practicalities should help clarify matters. I'll focus on situations involving short-term or acute care rather than long-term treatment or end-of-life issues.

Consent and refusal: What the law requires

All states recognize certain situations in which the express consent of the patient, either written or verbal, isn't necessary. Unless there is reason to believe the patient would refuse treatment, consent is implied in a medical emergency where there is immediate danger to the patient's life or health. And, for routine, basic care—X-rays, bathing, taking of vital signs, and the like—consent is implied by virtue of the patient's cooperation and presence in the hospital, clinic, or office.

Barring one of these exceptions, the long-held doctrine of *informed* consent applies. The patient must be told—in terms he can understand—all facts that a reasonably prudent patient would need to make an intelligent choice about treatment. This includes the nature and anticipated benefits of the proposed procedure or treatment, the alternatives, and the significant risks.

In a landmark case in 1980, the California Supreme Court decided that patients also have a right to be informed about the risks associated with *refusing* a recommended treatment or procedure.[1] Although the ruling only applied to California, it set a de facto national standard.

Provided the patient is competent and not a minor, he can either accept or reject the proposed course of care. However, that right isn't entirely absolute. Most states, for example, allow health care providers to provide life-saving emergency treatment in cases of attempted suicide even if the patient objects.

Other exceptions are more controversial, and are granted on an individual basis by the courts. When the patient is the sole support of young children, for instance, some courts have forced treatment on the parent to prevent abandonment of the children. Similarly, when treatment is necessary to protect a fetus—a C-section for an at-risk baby or drug rehabilitation for an addicted mother-to-be—some courts have mandated it. Other courts, however, have refused to do so.

The nurse's role in decision-making

Although the courts have overwhelmingly held that obtaining informed consent is the physician's responsibility, it's not uncommon for nurses to be involved in the process, by asking the patient to sign the consent form, for example. Nurses have a duty to notify the doctor—and advocate for the patient if necessary—if they believe the patient does not understand the treatment or procedure, has been coerced into agreeing to it, has changed his mind about it, or is incompetent.

As with informed consent, the courts have held that getting informed refusal is also the physician's duty. But two basic nursing responsibilities—patient education and advocacy—could be interpreted as imposing a legal burden on nurses to intervene when necessary. Keep in mind that patients who leave the hospital against medical advice (AMA) often do so when the treating physician is not present or quickly reachable. In such instances, it may be up to you to act.

Try to convince the patient to wait and speak with the doctor. If he won't, do what you can to make sure the patient's refusal of treatment is a truly informed one. Explain to him, in plain and simple terms, the consequences of leaving. For example: "Mr. Jones, your symptoms and tests indicate that you could be having a heart attack. If you are, your heart could stop beating very suddenly and without warning, and if that happens you could die."

Attempt to contact the physician as soon as possible. If feasible, try to uncover what's behind the patient's actions—it could be fear, frustration at having to wait for medical attention, or concern over the cost of treatment. Contact social services, the hospital chaplain, or any other service that might be able to help. Ask the patient for permission to contact a family member, who may be helpful in persuading the patient to accept medical advice.

Although as a nurse you can't make a legal determination as to whether a patient is competent to refuse treatment, you can and should assess his mental status. Evaluate whether he is alert and oriented to time, place, and person.

Be aware that from a legal perspective, patients are presumed to be competent to accept or refuse treatment—including those who are mentally ill, intoxicated, or have taken drugs. So any determination by health care providers to the contrary must be based on an individual assessment.

Be sure to document all relevant observations—such as the patient's statements and behavior—and communicate them to the physician. If the patient later sues, claiming his right to refuse treatment was violated, this could help demonstrate to a jury that there was a valid basis for the health care team's conclusions and actions.

Restraints should be used as a last resort. But if there's a reasonable belief that a patient is disoriented or incompetent, and leaving the hospital will immediately endanger his life, it may be appropriate to forcibly detain him.

Situations like this, which require the involvement of physicians and usually hospital administrators, are a legal catch-22: Not providing the treatment could lead to charges of negligence or abandonment; restraining the patient and providing treatment could result in charges of false imprisonment and battery.

Detailed charting is your safety net

It doesn't hurt to ask a competent adult who refuses treatment to sign an AMA form—in fact, most hospitals require that this be done—but a signature alone won't prove that an informed refusal took place. The key to that rests with your documentation in the medical record, which should paint a clear picture of the scenario that unfolded. Be sure to include the following:

- What the patient said, what you told the patient, and the patient's response. Use quotations whenever possible.
- A description of the patient's demeanor and behavior. Use objective, descriptive terms, not subjective words or opinions.
- A statement about the patient's mental status.
- Who you notified and when.

Here's an example of documentation that would give a plaintiff's attorney little to work with:

6/26/96 8:30 a.m.

8:15 a.m. Patient came out of his room and yelled, "I'm going home. I'm not staying for any more tests." Patient pounded fists on desk and shook his finger at staff. I told patient that his symptoms and tests indicated he may be having a heart attack, that if he left the hospital his heart could stop beating suddenly and without warning, and that if that happened he could die.

Patient listened, and then stated, "I'm leaving anyway." I placed a call to Dr. Smith at 8:17 a.m. Spoke with his assistant Mary Davis and left message. Notified nursing supervisor Gail Murphy of above. Patient gathered his belongings and left at 8:20 a.m. Patient was alert and oriented to time, place, and person before, during, and after this incident. (Nurse's Signature)

If there's time and the patient is receptive, you can try providing special discharge instructions—for instance, what the patient should and shouldn't do in his condition, what signs and symptoms warrant an immediate call to an ambulance. Document any instructions you provide. If the patient refused to sign an AMA form, document this as well.

What if the patient is a minor?

A different set of rules may apply if the patient is a child. In general, patients under the age of 18 cannot legally consent to or refuse treatment; a parent or guardian must do so for them. But you should be familiar with a few exceptions to this rule.

In most states, for instance, minors can consent to treatment for certain conditions, such as sexually transmitted diseases, pregnancy, and substance abuse.

"Emancipated" minors may be able to legally accept or refuse any treatment. The criteria needed to establish emancipation vary by state, but these are usually minors who are married, have a child, or are financially self-supporting. Emancipated minors are either defined by state statute or declared emancipated through court adjudication.

"Mature" minors may also be able to give or withhold consent. These are generally youths near the age of 18 who exhibit mature behavior in the eyes of a court or as defined by state law.

Unless one of these exceptions applies, treating a minor in a non-emergency situation without the consent of the parent or guardian could lead to charges of battery. However, parents and guardians generally don't have the authority to refuse life-saving, emergency treatment on behalf of their minor child for any reason—including religious convictions.

Your role as patient advocate makes the health of the child your first priority. Don't let the child leave the hospital without a parent or guardian. Immediately alert the physician and your supervisor any time a family's decision to refuse or stop treatment for their child could cause him harm. Disagreements over medical care can sometimes be mediated in the hospital—the ethics committee may be helpful in this regard. In some cases, though, a court order may be required to get the child the necessary treatment.

When a patient refuses appropriate medical treatment, ask yourself whether you did all that you could as an educator and an advocate. A Yes answer may not make it any easier to watch the patient walk out the hospital door. However, it should ease your conscience—and reduce your likelihood of being sued—if he later needs to be wheeled back in.

REFERENCES

1. Truman v. Thomas, 611 P.2d 902 (Cal. 1980).

Small patients, big legal risks

Societal changes and special situations that apply only to minors complicate all the usual liability issues when your patient is a child.

When a child is seriously ill or injured, emotions run high among relatives and caregivers alike. Even a routine hospitalization can cause extreme stress among family members. The sudden loss of control and strong emotions cause many adults to become extremely anxious about matters involving their child's treatment—and less accepting if there is a mistake.

Unless this volatile mix of emotions is managed properly, the stage is set for a lawsuit should a clinical mishap occur. And unless you are well-versed in the legal issues pertaining to children, you leave yourself and your institution open to liability.

Nurses working in pediatric units aren't the only RNs who are vulnerable. Those in hospital EDs, emergency clinics, home care, and other settings where children are treated could also find themselves in legal hot water if they're not prepared.

The way you relate can make the difference

Establishing rapport with the patient and family can reduce the likelihood that they will pursue legal action even if problems do arise. Quite simply, it's harder to sue someone who has been caring and helpful than someone you think is indifferent.

The most effective way to connect with the family is also one of the easiest: listen. A common complaint of parents who litigate is that no one took the time to really pay attention to them. Listening carefully to parents, and even seeking their advice, can pay off clinically, too. Seemingly insignificant clues—a change in the intensity or pitch of a child's cry, for instance—can signal a problem to a parent before any clinical symptoms appear.

When parents come to you with a seemingly minor concern or complaint, take it seriously. If it is a procedural problem, pass it on to the appropriate administrator. If it relates to the child's clinical condition, notify the attending physician or the nursing supervisor and chart it—"Mother states that patient appears unusually listless," for instance. Reassure the family that the concern will be investigated promptly, and document its resolution.

Don't assume everything is okay, though, just because parents don't approach you; some may be reluctant to air their concerns. To avoid or diffuse frustrations, ask parents whether they need anything or have any concerns they would like to discuss. Encourage communication between the health care team and the family.

Tackling the problem before a lawyer does

Be alert, too, to signs of a lawsuit waiting to happen. For example, if you overhear a parent complain that no one has checked to make sure an asthmatic child's bronchodilator is working, immediately inform the appropriate caregiver, who should then check the child's condition and reassure the parent.

If the situation deteriorates and the parent talks about seeing a lawyer, pass that information on to your supervisor or risk management department right away. The hospital's patient ombudsman, social worker, or risk manager can then approach the family and ask whether anything can be done for them. This early intervention may prevent a minor problem from escalating into a major issue.

Because parents may not always be around when routine care is given—or may not realize that a nurse who walks into the room is actually monitoring the patient—reinforce your care by keeping them thoroughly informed throughout their child's hospital stay. In the event of a clinical mistake—even if no serious injury results—inform parents of the incident right away so they are not caught off guard when they visit.

Choose your words carefully, to avoid alarming them: Telling parents their child was given too large a dose of medication will be less upsetting to them than using the word "overdose." You may wish to consult with your institution's risk manager on the best way to deliver unpleasant messages. Whatever words you use, though, it's vital to be honest and straightforward.

The statute of limitations: Buttressing your defense

Adult patients usually have a very limited period of time in which to initiate a malpractice suit: generally no more than four years after the alleged incident or after they become aware of the event. But most states allow an extended period of time for pediatric patients or family members acting on their behalf to file claims, often as long as a year beyond the state's legal age of majority.

Even after a claim is filed, the case may drag on for years more. If the incident in dispute occurred when the patient was born, a health care worker who is called as a trial witness may find herself testifying more than 20 years after the event.

Time is not the only problem. More claims arise from "routine" nursing tasks such as administering meds than from unique events that are likely to stand out in your memory. So in cases involving newborns or pediatric patients, thorough documentation that follows nursing policy and clearly identifies problems, nursing interventions, and resolutions takes on added importance.

Be sure that your facility does its part, too: The medical records department should have a long-term retention policy for preserving, in its original form, material on pediatric patients that could one day be used as evidence. The same retention policy should apply to X-rays, specimens, lab results, and other medical reports.

The murky waters of informed consent

With divorce, remarriage, single parenting, teenage pregnancies, and foster parenting, a growing number of children live in nontraditional households. Between 1970 and 1989, for instance, the proportion of children in the United States living with both parents dropped from 85% to 73%.[1] That makes it increasingly difficult to determine who has the authority to consent to or refuse treatment for a pediatric patient.

If the child's parents are married to each other or have joint custody, usually either spouse can sign the consent form or make treatment decisions. If divorce results in a sole custody arrangement, then generally the custodial parent is assumed to be the party who can give consent.

Such issues are always state-specific, however, and there are important exceptions to the general rules. In Georgia, for example, a court ruled that a do not resuscitate (DNR) order for a minor could not be implemented without the consent of both parents. Children may also have court-appointed guardians— who have the right to agree to treatment—instead of or in addition to parents.

Rules governing the confidentiality of patient information are also state-specific. For example, some states allow minors to seek treatment for substance abuse, sexually transmitted diseases, or rape without the knowledge or consent of their parents. When in doubt about to whom you should and shouldn't be talking, consult with your supervisor or risk manager. Refer anyone requesting a copy of the patient's chart to the medical records department.

Because of the complex legal issues involved, most hospitals do not expect nurses to determine who makes treatment decisions. When such questions arise, consult with your institution's risk manager. The admitting staff should also identify the party with the authority to give informed consent for a pediatric patient, and list the name of that person on the admitting document, which will become a part of the patient's chart.

If there are any questions or a family member disputes the authority of the designated individual, nurses should contact the admitting office rather than trying to resolve the issue on their own.

The person authorized to pick up the child at discharge should also be identified at the time of admission. This information should also appear on the admitting form that accompanies the patient's chart. Getting that information is one way to reduce the chances that a child will be abducted from the hospital—a possibility that all hospital nurses need to be aware of.

Speaking up if you suspect child abuse

Every state requires nurses and physicians to report cases of suspected child abuse.[2] Failing to do so, for whatever reason, endangers your patient and could put you in legal jeopardy as well.

Most states grant immunity from liability to those who report suspected child abuse, even if an investigation of the allegations reveals that no abuse has taken place—as long as the allegations were made in good faith. That does not guarantee that family members won't sue, but it does make it highly unlikely that you will be found liable for damages. Of course, the law will not protect a caregiver who files a report of child abuse when she has no reason to suspect it, or who does so with malicious intent.

Despite the emotional nature of child abuse, you must remain objective when assessing the patient's condition and documenting what you see. Chart facts, observations, and information received from the patient or parent, identifying the source of subjective statements—"Patient (or mother) states that ...," for example. Do not chart assumptions or speculate as to the cause or circumstances of the injuries.

Procedures for reporting suspected child abuse vary according to state statute and hospital policy. Regardless of how your institution elects to handle this delicate issue, it is vitally important that you know and follow the policies and procedures of your facility.

Awareness and anticipation are the watchwords when it comes to caring for pediatric patients. Placing the needs of child and family first greatly reduces your risk of liability. Knowing the laws that affect the way you practice and understanding the way the legal system operates is the surest way to avoid pitfalls and preventable mistakes.

REFERENCES

1. Weiler, K., & Helms, L. B. (1992). Who's in charge? Guardianships and children. MCN; American Journal of Maternal Child Nursing, 17(5), 232.
2. Fiesta, J. (1992). Protecting children: A public duty to report. Nursing Management, 23(7), 14.

Shedding some light on psychiatric care issues

A disturbed patient can complicate care and increase your risk of liability.

P atients with serious mental illness occupy more hospital beds than those with any other disease.[1] Suicide is the ninth leading cause of death in the United States and the third leading cause among those between the ages of 15 and 24.[2]

With statistics like these, nurses in all settings must know how to recognize patients with psychiatric or emotional disturbances and meet their special needs. Because caring for these patients can present special issues—in terms of safety and constitutional rights—nurses must also know what legal risks are involved and how to minimize them.

Protecting your patients from self-inflicted harm

Health care providers have been found liable in cases where patients that they knew—or should have known—to be suicidal injured or killed themselves. Providers can incur liability for suicides committed either in the hospital or outside it, if the patient should have been prevented from leaving the facility but wasn't.

The best way to prevent a patient from harming himself— and, in turn, protecting yourself and your employer from malpractice charges—is to identify those at risk for suicide and to take the necessary precautions to protect them.

To that end, be sure to assess each and every patient's mental health and try to identify those who may be thinking of suicide. If your patient appears depressed, question him further: Has he had thoughts of suicide? Does he have any specific plans to harm himself?

If he expresses suicidal thoughts, document it and inform his physician or a psychiatrist immediately. Do the same if you notice any worrisome changes in his behavior during the course of his care—changes in his sleep pattern or eating habits, for instance.

If, after consulting with the physician or psychiatrist, you are still worried about your patient's safety, recommend placing him under one-to-one observation, requiring a provider to check on him every 15 minutes, moving him closer to the nurses station, or any variation of supervision that you feel is needed given the circumstances. If your recommendations fall on deaf ears, take your concerns up the chain of command.

Any time a patient poses a threat to himself, inspect the areas that are accessible to him and remove potentially dangerous objects—scissors, breakable drinking glasses, cleaning products, belts, shoelaces, and so on. In extreme cases, you may even need to remove furniture from the patient's room.

The consequences of failing to provide a safe environment for a suicidal patient can be tragic. In one case, a patient was admitted to a psychiatric unit after slitting his wrists. Four days later he used a plastic garbage can liner to suffocate himself. Hospital records indicated that employees had performed as many as a dozen bed checks after he died; yet his suicide wasn't discovered until the next morning when an employee attempted to wake him. A Pennsylvania jury awarded the patient's widow $1.6 million.[3]

Protecting the patient may also mean restricting unsupervised access to seemingly innocuous places: In one suicide case, a patient waiting on line to shave in a hospital laundry washroom jumped into an uncovered vat of boiling liquid soap.

Make sure, too, that other caregivers know about the patient's psychiatric status. If a patient who was admitted after attempting suicide must temporarily go off your unit—say, to radiology—follow your facility's policy for notifying the staff in that area about his mental status and his need for supervision.

Finally, don't forget to document your assessment, your patient checks, and all pertinent statements made by the patient. Even if you see no reason to suspect that your patient could harm himself, it's still a good idea to chart his psychiatric status. Doing so could help demonstrate to a jury later why closer supervision was not provided.

Treating a patient against his will

Just because a patient has a psychiatric illness doesn't mean he's legally incompetent to make medical decisions. So, you're holding a two-edged sword: If you detain, restrain, or medicate a disturbed patient without his informed consent, you could wind up facing claims of false imprisonment and battery. But, if you don't detain a patient who poses a threat to himself or others you could be found liable for malpractice.

Because of the legal risks of both actions, you'll need to carefully weigh your patient's right to make decisions about his own care against your own concern for his or another person's safety. The medical and psychiatric staff should be involved in any decisions to involuntarily detain a patient, but if there's no time to consult them you will need to rely on your own nursing judgment.

Use restraints as a last resort and only to the degree reasonably necessary to keep the patient from injuring himself or others. Follow your hospital's restraint policy and document the specific behavior or statements that necessitated the application of restraints. Use objective terms when documenting and, whenever possible, quote the patient.

Be sure you know what state requirements have to be satisfied before detaining any patient against his will, and follow those protocols to the letter. A case heard before a California appeals court in 1996 highlights how important that can be:

A young man came to Southwood Psychiatric Center with his parents after telling his mother that he needed help. There he became combative, threatening to harm himself, his family, and the staff. Believing that he was dangerous, the staff physically restrained him when he tried to leave the facility.[4]

Soon after and pursuant to doctor's orders, a psychiatric nurse evaluated the young man and concluded that he had a mental disorder and was a threat to himself and others. She determined that he met the criteria—as outlined by state law—for a 72-hour hold and completed the necessary form to admit him.

Furthermore, the nurse documented her own and the staff's observations of the patient's behavior. She also read him a "Detainment Advisement" and advised him of his rights as an involuntary patient. Later that evening, with the patient still in restraints and highly agitated, she administered the tranquilizer Ativan.

After his release, the patient filed a lawsuit, charging the nurse and Southwood with, among other things, false imprisonment and battery.

The court rejected his claims. It found that the nurse and her employer had fully complied with state law and therefore could not be held liable. It also ruled that the administration of Ativan was reasonable: It was the only practical measure to protect the patient from harming himself and others.

Warning others of potential danger

Divulging information that a patient has told you in confidence can lead to allegations that you breached your duty to maintain confidentiality. But if your silence could endanger the life of another, failing to reveal information may also lead to liability.

The exception to the rule of confidentiality gained attention more than 20 years ago: A patient killed a woman named Tatiana Tarasoff after telling his therapist of his intention to do so. The therapist had made no attempt to inform the victim directly of the patient's plans. In its landmark ruling in this case, the California Supreme Court held that doctors and psychotherapists have a duty to warn intended victims.[5]

You should keep in mind, however, that the extent to which a provider has a duty to warn varies: As in the California case, a provider's duty may extend to any person threatened by his patient if such a warning is essential to prevent that person from being harmed. Or, it could extend to those who are reasonably foreseeable victims of the patient's dangerous propensities, not just those who the patient specifically identified.

So, be sure you're familiar with the law in the states where you practice. If your patient tells you he's going to hurt someone, or you hear him telling someone else that, take it seriously and question the patient. If you find that the threat has merit, you may not have to warn the intended victim personally; but you do have to inform the psychiatrist and your supervisor immediately. Also document the threat in the patient's chart.

There's no question that mental and emotional problems can complicate the care you provide. But carefully listening to and observing your patients, providing them with a safe environment, and knowing what the law expects will help you provide the best care possible—and keep you out of legal trouble.

REFERENCES

1. National Alliance for the Mentally Ill. (1994). Mental illness: Information for writers. Arlington, VA: Author.
2. Rosenberg, H. M., Ventura, S. J., et al. (1996, October). Births and deaths: United States, 1995. Monthly vital statistics report, 45(3, Suppl. 2), 31.
3. Lewis, L. (Ed.). (1996). Pennsylvania man used garbage can liner to commit suicide. Medical Malpractice Verdicts, Settlements & Experts, 12(1), 43.
4. Heater v. Southwood Psychiatric Center, 49 Cal. Rptr. 2d 880 (1996).
5. Tarasoff v. The Regents of the University of California, 13 Cal. 3d 177, 529 P.2d 553 (1974).

Home care: More autonomy, more legal risks

As the economic advantages of home care become increasingly obvious, more and more nurses will be moving into that setting— and facing added responsibilities and legal risks.

One thing the relentless push for shorter hospital stays and less expensive care has accomplished is to push home care further into the mainstream. Hospitals and other health care facilities are touting the advantages of sending patients home as soon as possible.

Most nurses are aware that moving out of the hospital setting into home care will mean greater autonomy, but often they have little more than a vague idea of what that will mean. Here is a look at some of the situations you're likely to encounter, and tips on how to safeguard home care patients and sidestep legal risks.

When to go up the chain of command

Let's say that you have been caring for a patient who's had a stroke. One day you receive a frantic call from his wife, who thinks that he's had another one. You rush over, assess the patient, and find that his symptoms suggest a transient ischemic attack instead. Even though he is in somewhat better condition than you had anticipated, you do not want to leave without speaking to his physician, whom you suspect will want to examine the patient and possibly adjust the medication orders. But by the time you're ready to leave—and you are needed at another patient's home—the doctor still hasn't returned your calls.

Although many nurses who find themselves in this situation would not hesitate to contact another physician, many are uncertain about where they can turn for help. In fact, nursing administrators at home care agencies are often shocked to learn how few of their staffers actually know the chain of command.

Before starting out on a new assignment, a home care nurse should make sure the agency provides a list of telephone numbers to call in such situations and detailed instructions about proper procedures. Among the specifics it should address: When the attending physician cannot be reached, is it appropriate for the nurse to seek assistance from the department head or the chief of medicine at the hospital where the doctor has privileges? Under what sort of circumstances, if any, should a direct call be placed to the medical director of the home care agency?

Nonclinical emergencies should be covered as well: What action should be taken if a family member of an acutely ill patient threatens to harm you if you enter the house, for instance, or if you visit a homebound patient and find her alone with no food, money, or medication? No matter what the hierarchy at a particular agency, someone—an administrator or clinical supervisor—should be on call seven days a week, 24 hours a day, to consult and advise in such situations.

If a patient's condition is rapidly deteriorating, however, no nurse is likely to hesitate to do whatever is necessary to get proper medical treatment. In a situation like the one with the stroke patient, you should probably not wait around any longer for the doctor to call. You need to get the patient to an ED, since TIA can precede stroke. Invoke your chain of command and request an ambulance. In a life-threatening situation, call EMS, of course. A final word of warning: No matter whom you call to report a significant change or to discuss your patient's condition, in home care—as in hospital care—documentation is the key to legal protection. Note every attempt to reach the attending physician, the time and content of the messages left, the facts conveyed in each conversation, and any efforts you have made to go further up the chain of command—whom you spoke to and what was said.

If equipment failure jeopardizes your patient

Suppose your patient has chronic obstructive pulmonary disease and is on a portable ventilator. You check the flow rate on each visit, but one day your patient complains that he has been frequently waking up with a headache. You are afraid the ventilator is improperly calibrated and wonder whether the patient's receiving too much oxygen.

Any time that you care for a patient who is on special equipment, you must be thoroughly familiar with it. You have got to know how to operate the equipment, monitor it, provide associated care—such as suctioning—and detect potential problems. If you are assigned a patient whose care involves the use of a device you're unfamiliar with, insist on getting the proper training beforehand. And refuse to accept an assignment if you feel you are not qualified to give the specialized care required. For example, if the patient is an ostomate who is suffering from acute constipation, and you do not know how to irrigate the colon using the traditional equipment, do not take the case.

You are responsible, too, for making sure that the patient or his caregivers know how to operate any equipment used in the home. Ideally, you should provide them with written instructions detailing what to do if an alarm sounds or other problems arise, review the procedures carefully in person, and request a return demonstration. Document in the chart all teaching that you have given to the patient and family members. If equipment failure could be life-threatening, as in the case of a malfunctioning ventilator, be sure there is back-up equipment in the home or a phone number to call—usually provided by the supplier—for emergency service or replacement.

If you will be using any of your own equipment, such as a sphygmomanometer, get written approval to do so. Because agencies typically require evidence that equipment is in proper order before they will give such permission, having their go-ahead can protect you from liability if a problem arises. If you have reason to suspect that a piece of equipment is either inaccurate or malfunctioning, as in the example with the ventilator, call for emergency service and then immediately report the problem to your supervisor. Your agency should also have a written policy on file for reporting equipment failure. Any sort of equipment-related injury must be noted in the medical record as well as documented on an incident report.

If a malfunction causes serious injury, illness, or death, you're obligated under the Safe Medical Devices Act of 1990 (SMDA) to report the occurrence to the FDA and to the equipment manufacturer within 10 weekdays. You should describe the suspected malfunction and provide relevant details about the patient's condition and the event. This information must be kept confidential, and it cannot be used against you or your agency in any subsequent legal proceedings.[1]

Ideally, if you think a piece of equipment isn't working properly—whether the situation is life-threatening or not—you should remain with the patient until the equipment has been fixed, replaced, or its use is discontinued by the physician.

When to worry about informed consent

What do you do if you find yourself in this situation: You are visiting a 37-year-old cancer patient for the first time. She is anemic and requires weekly blood transfusions. You are qualified and prepared to perform the procedure in her home. But there is nothing in the patient's chart to indicate that she has been informed of the benefits and risks, or that she has consented to the transfusions. If the patient's willing, should you go ahead and give the blood anyway? Traditionally, it's been up to the clinician who is performing a procedure to obtain informed consent; until recently, that has almost always been the physician. But as potentially risky procedures like blood transfusions or the insertion of peripherally inserted central catheters (PICCs) have become increasingly common in outpatient settings, more and more nurses perform them without the close supervision of physicians.

Home care nurses are, in fact, in uncharted legal waters when it comes to the question of consent. While several recent court rulings have made it clear that nurses giving immunizations in an outpatient setting have a duty to obtain consent from their patients,[2] no such duty has been established for home care nurses.

Thus far, no nurse or home care agency has been brought to court for failing to obtain consent, nor has consent obtained by a nonphysican been ruled invalid.[3] However, you would be wise to go ahead and obtain consent rather than run the risk of the patient suffering ill effects and afterwards claiming she didn't understand what was being done to her.

With few clear-cut guidelines to follow, attorneys often advise both the physician who orders an invasive procedure and the nurse who performs it to obtain written authorization. If a nurse enters a patient's home and finds that informed consent has not been documented, the RN should attempt to contact the physician to determine whether consent was obtained and then go ahead and get written consent herself. For a consent to be legally valid, the nurse must be fully trained and competent to carry out the procedure in question, the patient must be informed of the associated benefits and risks, and the nurse must be acting within the bounds of her state nurse practice act.

Keeping patients fully informed also means advising them of their right to refuse treatment under the Patient Self-Determination Act (PSDA), including a DNR option. It is your legal obligation to document their wishes and, when necessary, to make sure their family members and other health care providers are aware of them as well.

What to consider when you delegate

Home care nurses often supervise aides who provide daily unskilled care for patients the RNs see on a weekly basis. Suppose that one morning the phone rings and an aide across town tells you that an elderly patient she was helping out of bed has fallen and fractured his hip. The patient has already been transported to the hospital, the aide explains to you, but the family is angry and they are threatening to sue. Could you be a target of that lawsuit, too?

You could be indeed. As a supervisor, you are responsible for making sure that an employee who is working under you—in this case, the aide—has proper training and adequate supervision. It is also up to you to assure that the duties she performs fall within the scope of that training.

In this particular instance, because aides routinely reposition patients and assist them in and out of bed, it's unlikely that you'd be liable for the actions of the aide. To prevent an aide from exceeding her authority and performing procedures that could get her—and you—into legal trouble, discuss the proper care for each patient she's assigned, and clarify the circumstances under which you are to be called. Provide written parameters whenever possible: An aide caring for a child with pneumonia might be told to call if respirations exceed 35 per minute, for instance. Review the patient's care plan: Make sure it's followed, and that the aide thoroughly documents her actions. Again, complete and accurate records represent your best defense against a malpractice claim.

REFERENCES

1. Brent, N. J. (1992). High—tech care and medical devices: The Safe Medical Devices Act of 1990. Home Healthcare Nurse, 10(3), 11.
2. Sweeney, M. L. (1991). Your role in informed consent. RN, 54(8), 55.
3. Staff. (1993). Documentation, training protect hospitals from risk in home care. Hospital Risk Management, 15(11), 164

Q&A:
Patient Care Issues

The Risks of "Nursing" Your Friends' Kids

As a pediatric nurse, friends often ask me about their children's health problems. I don't mind giving out general advice, but I feel uncomfortable when they ask me to "take a look at" their child. What are the liability risks if I do?

Considerable. If you evaluate a child and then give the parent your opinion about that child's health, you are making a medical diagnosis—and usually without the benefit of a complete history or a comprehensive physical examination.

If you misdiagnose the problem and the child comes to harm as a result, you could be sued for malpractice. And, unless you have private malpractice insurance, you'll have no coverage; your employer's carrier won't cover you because you were acting outside the scope of your employment.

The best response to give your friends is to call the pediatrician's office and discuss the matter with the doctor or nursing staff.

When patients self-administer medications

A doctor at my hospital sometimes allows patients to keep sleeping pills they've brought from home. I'm afraid that a patient will forget to tell the nurses about any pills they've taken, or that they'll take too many. Who is liable if a patient overdoses?

The doctor. Allowing a patient to keep pills of any kind not only violates the usual and customary standard of care but also goes against common sense. If the patient overdoses, the hospital may be liable as well—for having a doctor who fails to conform to customary standards on its medical staff.

You should make a written report to your supervisor informing her of this physician's practice, and if necessary, take your concern up the chain of command.

Nursing care shouldn't be a family affair

A nurse at the small, rural hospital where I work was assigned to care for her cousin after a snow storm left our unit short-staffed. Is it legal for a nurse or doctor to care for a family member?

In most cases, it's not illegal for a health care provider to care for a family member, except in certain narrowly defined circumstances. For example, a patient's nurse or physician generally cannot be his health care proxy as well. And in some states, physicians can't prescribe controlled substances for family members.

Nonetheless, caring for a family member isn't wise, particularly if the patient's condition is serious. The nurse's clinical judgment could become clouded by emotions. And there's also the potential for a conflict of interest. If the patient dies and leaves money to the nurse-relative who cared for her, for instance, the nurse's motives and actions might be called into question.

If patients ask what you think about a doctor

One of the orthopedists I work with doesn't respond to calls and misses signs and symptoms that seem apparent to me. When a patient asked my opinion of the doctor, I dodged the question because I was afraid of being sued for defamation. Was I correct to be concerned?

Defamation means that you publicly communicated something that you knew—or should have known—to be false and harmful to a person's good name or reputation. If your suspicions about the doctor were reasonable and you answered the patient's question honestly, it's unlikely that a defamation suit would have been successful.

Practically speaking, though, a forthright answer could put you in an awkward position, since you have to work with the doctor. I suggest you steer patients who have similar questions in the right direction, without answering them directly. For example, ask the patient what specifically is worrying her, state that those concerns seem valid, and suggest that she seek another doctor's opinion.

There's something else you should do, too: If you suspect the doctor is incompetent or dangerous, you have a professional obligation to report that fact to your supervisor or state licensing board in accordance with state law.

When patients leave the ED before treatment

I work in a busy ED, where patients who don't have life-threatening symptoms often have to wait hours before being treated. I worry about patients who get tired of waiting and leave. Could I be accountable if one of them becomes seriously ill because they didn't receive medical attention?

Yes, if the delay in treatment was unwarranted or the patient was not informed of the risks of leaving. And you'll need to be able to demonstrate that you acted appropriately on both counts.

Re-evaluate ED patients at reasonable intervals and document their status each time. This will show that you were monitoring the patient throughout his stay. If a patient wants to leave before being treated, tell him the risks and document that you have done so. If he still wants to go, ask him to sign an Against Medical Advice form, and file it in his chart. If he refuses to sign, document this in the chart as well.

Giving meds without MD orders

Under a new hospital protocol, nurses are to administer designated categories of oral meds pre-procedure to patients who are NPO, unless contraindicated by physician order. I'm concerned about the risks of this policy. Shouldn't the doctor specifically order what medications nurses are to administer?

Standing orders are not uncommon, and may be legitimate for patient care purposes. However, the policy you describe sounds like a dangerous one from a legal standpoint, one that exposes physicians, nurses, and the hospital to easily avoidable liability. The problem lies in the fact that a nurse could easily interpret silence on the physician's part to mean that the medications should be given, when in fact, the physician may simply have failed to review the patient's drugs and write an order holding one or more of them.

Since the physician should be reviewing the medication list before a patient's procedure anyway, it would be just as easy—and more foolproof—to have the doctor order the medications that are to be given, instead of any that should be withheld. I suggest that you talk to your facility's risk manager about changing the policy.

Who's held responsible for equipment failure?

A malfunctioning ventilator recently caused a fire at my hospital and one patient was injured as a result of smoke inhalation. Could any of the nurses be held liable?

Yes, if the patient is able to prove any of the following: the malfunction should have been detected by a nurse but wasn't; the ventilator alarms were turned off; a nurse did not respond to an audible alarm or a call for help from the patient in a timely fashion; or a nurse failed to set up or use the ventilator in accordance with the hospital's policy and the manufacturer's instructions.

In addition, regardless of the cause of the fire, a nurse may be found negligent if she failed to follow the hospital's policy and procedure for fires.

When you leave one patient to help another

I was giving a patient a sponge bath when the woman in the next bed started choking. I rushed to help without first putting up the siderail on my patient's bed. When she leaned over to see what was happening, she fell out. Legally, am I at fault?

Even though the situation was an urgent one, a lawyer could argue that you were negligent because you failed to anticipate and avoid an easily preventable occurrence involving a patient over whom you had direct and immediate control. He would have an even stronger case if the patient required siderail protection, for example because she was elderly, confused, or medicated.

Your actions after the accident could be important, too. After taking care of both patients, you should have discussed the events with your supervisor or risk manager. All relevant details should have been charted—for example, the fact that you instructed the first patient not to move. Hopefully, you gave yourself time to calm down before you charted. It's easy to forget important facts when you're distressed.

If parents watch when kids receive care

When children come to our ED, their parents are allowed to watch as the staff provides care. When they become upset or agitated, though, my attention gets distracted from the patient. What are the legal risks of having parents present while their kids are being treated?

Visibly upset or distraught parents may hinder the patient's treatment, and even harm themselves or a staff member if they lose control. Depending on the circumstances, you and your employer could be held responsible for any resulting injury.

However, because parents are usually able to calm and reassure their children while maintaining self-control, the benefits of having them present generally outweigh the risks. To minimize the likelihood that parents will become overly upset, procedures should be briefly explained to them beforehand if time permits, or during the treatment itself.

If parents do become extremely upset, they should be told in a kind but firm manner that their behavior is distracting the staff or upsetting their child, and they must wait in another part of the ED. If their behavior becomes aggressive or they have to be phys̲ː ̲ ̲ removed from the treatment area, document the incident report.

Failing to heed doctor's orders

A nurse on my unit withheld several doses of a scheduled medication without notifying the attending physician. What legal risks did she take?
The nurse could be subject to disciplinary action by both her employer and the state board of nursing for professional misconduct. What's more, intentionally failing to carry out a doctor's order can be construed as the unlawful practice of medicine, which is not only grounds for a lawsuit, but, in some states, a criminal act punishable by jail time. Finally, if the patient suffered an injury because he did not receive the medication, he could sue bring a malpractice suit.

Deciding whether a particular order is appropriate is an important nursing function; one you perform every day. And there may indeed be circumstances when a nurse should refuse to carry out an order. That's why hospitals have an established chain of command and specific policies and procedures for nurses to follow when they have a valid basis for questioning a physician's order.

When doctors disagree

At the small ED where I work, a stat X-ray reading is done by a staff radiologist, then we send the X-ray out to a radiology group for a final reading. What should we do when the two readings differ?
Notify the patient about the disagreement. Your facility should have an established procedure for contacting patients about second readings and documenting that this has been done. If it doesn't, talk to your risk manager or administrator about developing one.

To prevent patients from becoming angry—and filing suits—be up front with them when the X-ray is first read. Tell them that the findings are initial, and that a second radiologist will be looking at the X-ray as well, usually within 24 hours.

Going over your supervisor's head

When a nursing home patient I was caring for developed serious cardiovascular symptoms, I notified the DON. I thought a transfer to a hospital was necessary, but the nursing director summarily ruled against it. What was my duty in this situation?

If the DON ruled against the transfer without even consulting a physician, she made a medical judgment and was therefore acting beyond the scope of her authority. In fact, she could be charged with practicing medicine without a license.

Your role is clear-cut: If you believe a patient needs immediate medical attention, you are obligated to see that she gets it. In the situation you describe, you should have called the attending physician and informed him of your clinical findings. If he didn't authorize the care you felt was necessary, you should have gone to the medical director, and then up the chain of command if necessary.

Whenever you need to do so, document your actions in the patient's chart. As always, state facts, not conclusions.

Can referrals get you in hot water?

At our clinic we frequently make referrals to outside facilities. Are there any liability risks involved?

Yes. If the referral is part of the patient's care, such as a referral to an oncologist after a suspicious finding, the patient's health care team must make sure she understands the possible seriousness of her condition and the need for the referral. If she doesn't and fails to make an appointment as a result, they may well be liable.

Liability can also result on another score: If clinic personnel refer patients to health care providers who they know are unqualified or provide substandard care.

Communicating with the hearing impaired

When I had to give discharge instructions to a deaf patient recently, a family member told me to ask his sister to convey what I said in sign language. Is that proper?
Never make assumptions about the needs of hearing-impaired patients; ask them, in writing if necessary, how they want to communicate. Under the Americans with Disabilities Act (ADA) of 1990 and the Rehabilitation Act of 1973, hospitals must offer reasonable accommodations for hearing-impaired patients—providing qualified interpreters and auxiliary tools like teletype machines, for example.

Health care institutions—like other public facilities—are expected to provide the method of assistance that the patient chooses, unless doing so would impose financial hardship or an undue burden.

It's fine to have a patient's relative use sign language to interpret, if that's what he wishes. But be aware that any time a third party relays information, there's the possibility that something will be omitted. As a backup, give the patient written instructions to take home, too.

Discretion in the ED

I work in a busy, crowded emergency room, and we get our share of patients who've been drinking or using drugs. Can I question patients about possible alcohol or drug use in front of other patients?
There's no specific legal prohibition against it. But because patients have a right to privacy and confidentiality from the moment they arrive in the ED, you shouldn't be questioning them in front of others—no matter what type of information you're inquiring about.

An exception would be if asking in public is medically necessary and can't be avoided—if, for example, you're doing triage and the patient appears to need immediate treatment. If that's not the case, take the patient to a private room before you take a history.

Keep comments out of earshot of patients

A nurse on my unit makes remarks about a patient's condition at the bedside when that patient is sleeping. I'm concerned that the comments will somehow register with the patient or that a roommate will overhear. What are the ramifications if that happens?

The old adage, "Loose lips sink ships" applies here. If the roommate overhears, the nurse is vulnerable to a breach of confidentiality claim. If the nurse signed a pledge of confidentiality when she was hired, a breach of that agreement could be grounds for her dismissal.

And you are right to be concerned about the effect of the remarks on the patient himself. It's been shown that patients under anesthesia can remember comments made in the OR. The same could happen with a patient who is sleeping.

Remind this nurse about the possible impact of her remarks and tactfully suggest that she limit her comments to more appropriate settings.

Get consent to divulge patient information

I work in a college health service clinic. A psychotic student was sent to the hospital and the college administration is now requesting information about the patient. Am I violating any confidentiality rules by complying with the request?

Quite possibly. Patient confidentiality is highly protected by law, but there are exceptions. In the case you describe, a breach of confidentiality is warranted if the patient poses a serious danger to himself or another person. However, the information can be divulged only to parties with a legitimate need to know, such as other members of the health care team, a potential victim, or the police. It's doubtful whether the college administration would fit into the "need-to-know" category, because it deals primarily with academic issues.

To avoid a breach of confidentiality claim, your school administration should ask hospitalized students—or their guardians if they are minors or judged incompetent—to sign a release-of-information form. This form should state what information is being requested, for what purposes, who will have access to it, and the time period for which the release is valid.

Unit Two:

Documentation and Administration

Documentation: Every word counts

Defensive charting is one of the surest ways to tip the scales of justice in your favor. Here are the basics.

From a legal standpoint, your documentation is just as important as the care you provide. A recent case proves this point nicely: A young man had developed respiratory distress after what should have been a routine appendectomy. Despite intervention, respiratory arrest quickly followed. Resuscitation failed.

Shocked at such an unexpected death, the patient's family initiated a lawsuit. After reviewing the medical record, however, their attorney advised them to drop it. The hospital records made it clear that everything possible had been done for the patient, leaving no basis for a claim of negligence.

If that young man had been your patient, would your documentation have tipped the scales in your favor? Or would the record have been full of holes—with assessments noted but interventions omitted, perhaps, or a summary of actions that were taken but no indication that they were subsequently followed up? A review of some common charting deficiencies and a list of documentation do's and don'ts will help you keep your record-keeping on target.

The chart tells the patient's story

An attorney or a risk manager should be able to review a patient's medical record and reconstruct the care he received, even if months or years have passed. If key facts or notes on follow-up are missing from the record and the patient sues, it's hard for an attorney to mount a strong defense.

To be certain that your documentation is complete, address these three vital aspects of patient care: assessment, intervention, and patient response. Be particularly alert in the following instances, where charting gaps most commonly occur:

When vital signs are abnormal. Any significant deviation from normal—whether it's fever, elevated BP, or slow respiration rate—demands a notation showing what is being done about it. If you notify the resident or attending physician, record the time you made the call, the doctor's response and whether you carried out his order. If you are unable to reach the doctor initially, note the time you received a return call, tried the call again, or contacted someone else.

If your response to abnormal findings is to monitor the patient more closely, specify that in the chart—and note whether the patient's condition improves or deteriorates. If his course is an up-and-down one, note how often change occurs.

When a patient codes. As in the case of the appendectomy patient, an unexpected bad outcome often results in a lawsuit. Documenting what happened during a code or other emergency is especially crucial, since plaintiffs' attorneys often argue that monitoring was inadequate and intervention too late.

Yet emergency situations are precisely when documentation is apt to fall short. To avoid charting gaps, many hospitals keep code sheets on crash carts. A member of the code team gets the job of checking off each intervention and jotting down the time that it's carried out. If your facility does not have such a procedure, talk to your supervisor and your risk manager about developing one.

Once a crisis is over, check the documentation to be sure it's complete. If the patient has been moved—to the ICU, for example—follow him there to review his chart and see that nothing crucial was omitted.

When a patient is transferred. Any patient move—from ED to ICU, OR to PACU, even from one med/surg unit to another—calls for a patient assessment. Document the condition of the patient soon after he arrives on your unit, and again right before he leaves. It should go without saying that the chart will contain a record of the patient's condition on admission to your institution, and that assessments are updated at the beginning and end of each shift.

Chart your interventions and those of others

To save charting time and space, make concise notations on routine tasks such as bathing a patient. Use forms and flow sheets when appropriate, but make certain that they provide a complete picture of what's going on.

When necessary, document any observations in detail. Note the color, consistency, and quantity of any drainage, for example. Describe the quantity of exudate or body fluid that can't be measured, such as vaginal blood: "blood the size of a quarter on one peripad," for example, is far clearer than "light bleeding."

Chart deficits, such as inactivity, lethargy, or lack of response. Describe non-compliant behavior. Use quotes to report any patient self-assessment as well.

To document nursing interventions, note protective measures, such as putting the side rails up, helping the patient to the bathroom, and advising her not to get out of bed unassisted. Document the use of specialized equipment or procedures—even something as simple as putting an eggcrate mattress on the bed. If the equipment is electrically powered, such as pneumatic compression cuffs, record the time of initial use. Chart offers of assistance from other hospital staffers, such as a visit from a chaplain or social worker, and whether they were accepted or declined.

Spell out instructions and discharge planning

Even though there have been few lawsuits brought alleging premature discharge, legal experts are expecting to see more of them as length of stay gets shorter and shorter. To defend against such suits, the record should demonstrate not only that a patient was well enough to be discharged home, but also that he and his family were given adequate preparation.

Note any handouts or written instructions that he received. Describe any patient teaching that you did; document comprehension by noting that the patient or a member of his family completed a satisfactory return demonstration.

Also chart any restrictions in activity, functional deficits, and conditions that warrant a call to the physician. If return visits have already been scheduled, include that information, as well.

Because discharge planning will, more than likely, be a joint, multi-departmental effort, it is a sensible plan for hospitals to keep this documentation separate—in the same file as the rest of the patient's medical record, but in a separate divider, perhaps. Copies of any referrals, summaries sent to the home health agency or other post-discharge providers, together with a tentative care plan, belong in the discharge folder as well.

Heed these charting do's and don'ts

To keep your patients' medical records clear, concise, and complete, here are a few additional reminders:

Do

- Restrict use of abbreviations to those that your administration has approved; get a list from the medical records department.
- Include the time, date, and your signature on each entry.
- Delete an entry by drawing a thin line through it, not by erasing or obliterating it. Make sure it's still legible.
- Follow your hospital policy regarding addendums; use them only if you have omitted a vital piece of information, and only within the prescribed time period.
- Draw a line to the end of a page or blank section on a chart, much as you would draw a line through a blank space on a check.

Don't

■ Use the chart to accuse or blame.

■ Draw unfounded conclusions. Don't write "patient fell," unless you witnessed the fall. Instead, describe only the facts you know for sure: "entered room, found patient on floor," for instance.

■ Characterize a patient with such words as "hostile" or "combative." Describe his behavior.

■ Make an addendum or change because you're afraid you'll look bad or you're afraid of liability.

Charting is an important part of nursing, and the best way to show that you have met the standard of care. When a crisis occurs, careful documentation can head off a lawsuit—or help your attorney mount a successful defense.

A lawyer's chart review

Here's what an attorney will look for when he or she reviews a medical record. Try doing a review from this perspective on your own charts to see if they'd pass muster.

Not too long ago, the only person who could freely access a patient's chart was the physician. In recent years, though, the medical record has become an increasingly public document, open to review not only by patients but also licensing agencies, accreditation bodies, hospital committees, insurers, attorneys, and jurors.

Malpractice insurance companies regularly review the medical records of patients at hospitals, clinics, and offices. And they invariably find problems.

The fact is that many nurses underestimate how crucial good documentation is in warding off or defending against a malpractice claim. And, understandably, they do not see what a medical record looks like through an attorney's eyes.

Here, we'll tell you *and* offer some guidelines that can protect you and your employer from liability. We'll also discuss the right way to document occurrences in an incident report.

The rules of thumb for safe charting

An attorney who's looking at a chart—whether your employer's counsel who's trying to determine if staffers are complying with good charting rules or a plaintiff's attorney trying to bolster his client's case—will ask key questions. To do a prospective review yourself, pull between 10 and 20 medical records to review. Ask the following questions:

Are all entries legible? An attorney reviewing charts is often faced with notes and even entire charts that can't be deciphered. Although bad penmanship may be the subject of jokes, it's no laughing matter in court. A number of cases have had to be settled because the provider who wrote the note couldn't read his own handwriting.

Are there grammatical or spelling errors? This seems like a minor point. But in litigation these mistakes can help a plaintiff's attorney discredit you, and make it difficult for your own attorney to portray you as an educated professional.

Is the language objective? All statements in the record should be based on facts, concrete observations, or the patient's own statements. Avoid vague and subjective documentation, such as "wound appears infected." Be specific instead—"wound mottled with green, foul-smelling discharge," for instance. Document by your senses—what you see, hear, smell, feel, and so on.

Are abbreviations only those that are commonly accepted? Charts frequently contain nonstandard abbreviations—for example, TWO (totally whacked out) to describe a patient who is disoriented. Such abbreviations could be misinterpreted by a patient and jury to indicate a lack of compassion and objectivity on the nurse's part.

Are entries signed correctly? Signatures should follow every chart entry, be legible, and include the first name or initial, last name, and professional identifier (RN, LPN, etc.). It may seem obvious to you who's written the note, but prevailing professional standards require a signature.

Are entries dated and timed? Check to see whether each note indicates the month, day, year (which in a lengthy chart can be difficult to determine), and time that the note was written. If the events being described happened at an earlier time, such as the start of a shift, that time should be indicated within the note.

Is the chart free of erasures and other alterations? Made innocently or not, alterations cast doubt on the writer's credibility and can render cases indefensible. Common examples include writing over an incorrect number, changing "L" to "R," scribbling out mistakes, and adding forgotten information to the margin of a note or squeezing it in between the lines of an existing note.

The proper way to correct a mistake is to draw a single line through the error, date and initial it, and continue your note. To add information to an existing entry, write the date and time of the new entry at the next available space and include: "Addendum to note of (date and time of prior note)."

Are all entries made in black or blue ink? We've all seen entries written with pencils, colored markers, and colored inks. While there's probably nothing illegal about that, it's not a good idea. Since pencil can be easily erased, the suggestion of tampering can be easily made. Besides, it's often necessary to make photocopies of a chart and pencil and many light colored inks don't copy well—leaving the recipient with a document that's difficult or impossible to read.

Are known allergies highlighted? One of the most difficult cases to defend is that of a patient who's been prescribed or given medication to which he has a documented allergy. For this reason, the fact that a patient has an allergy to a medication should be prominently displayed on a conspicuous part of the chart.

Be careful, however, that the allergy alert doesn't breach the patient's right to confidentiality. A red sticker on the chart, for example, could be used to remind providers to look at the patient's history; a sticker that boldly proclaims PENICILLIN ALLERGY might easily be seen by other patients when it's on a countertop or door. And that's a breach of confidentiality.

Are flow sheets filled out completely? All boxes or spaces on a flow sheet should be filled in—even if it's only with "N/A" to indicate items that are not applicable to that particular patient. Blank spaces raise doubts about whether something was or wasn't done.

Omissions in the record can be just as costly

Not only should you evaluate how things are documented, you also should check to see *what* is documented. The following information should be included:

- A patient's refusal of treatment or noncompliance. Documentation of the patient's role in the course of treatment is extremely important to the successful defense of a case. Avoid generalizations such as "patient uncooperative." Instead document specific behaviors that indicate the patient was noncompliant—his refusal to take a prescribed medication, for example, or to participate in an exercise regimen.

- Patient teaching. To avoid allegations that the patient was not fully advised of side effects, symptoms, when to seek further care, and the like, document all patient education and instructions you've given. An even better alternative to charting this information each time you give it is to use pre-printed instruction sheets; have the patient sign the sheet, then make a photocopy of it to keep in the chart. Or, use a two-part carbonless form and keep one copy. That way you have signed proof that you instructed the patient and exactly what was covered in the discussion, with minimal writing on your part.

And remember, any time you use an interpreter when instructing a patient, document who the interpreter was and that you had the patient's consent to convey confidential information through her.

- Telephone instructions or advice. This is one of the most crucial pieces of information to have in the chart from the defense perspective—and one of the most inconsistently documented by nurses working in EDs, labor and delivery, clinics, and offices. Without such documentation, it's often the patient's word against yours.

Make sure to record the date and time of the call, names of participants, and the substance of the conversation. If the advice was dispensed to someone for whom there was no patient chart, keep a record of the call in a log book.

■ Follow-up for test results. If results are misplaced or not promptly communicated and a delay in treatment results, liability usually rests at least partially with those who ordered the test. So any time test results aren't received in a timely manner, call the appropriate lab or department, find out why, and document that you have done so. If you work in an ED, clinic, or office and need to notify a patient about abnormal test results—such as misread X-rays—after he has left the premises, document this follow-up. Include the date and time, and the substance of the discussion.

The right way to document an incident

Although in some states incident reports are discoverable—when requested in litigation, they must be produced—they're primarily for internal use only. They're a crucial component in any risk management and quality improvement program.

The exact criteria for filling out an incident report varies by institution. But these reports are generally used when any unplanned or unusual event causes, or has the potential to cause, physical injury or property damage.

Whatever the nature of the incident, accurately record the particulars: the time and date it occurred, the patient's name, which family member was notified, at what time, and whether in person or by phone. Record the name of the doctor who was notified and the time the call was made.

Give an objective description of the incident, without pointing a finger at anyone—and that includes yourself. Use direct quotes to convey important details from other people, for example, the patient's description of why and how he fell out of bed. Be sure to include the patient's words in quotation marks and preface them with "Patient states ... ."

Also document your patient assessment. Use clinical terms and report what you see, hear, and feel, rather than what you surmise.

Be aware, however, that some incident reports actually require you to speculate; these forms include a question about what you think caused the incident. If that's the case, keep your answer concise and refer to the facts that led you to reach that conclusion.

Document any action you took in the immediate aftermath of the incident, like getting a patient who fell back into bed or obtaining orders for X-rays. Don't document follow-up care, however; that information belongs in the patient's chart.

In the chart, you'll record many of the same facts you put in the incident report: when the incident occurred, a brief factual description, patient assessment, notification of family and physician, and treatment rendered. Do not make reference to filling out an incident report; by doing so, you could be making a plaintiff's attorney aware of its existence.

No matter what type of information you're documenting, always strive for clarity, completeness, and professionalism. It's one of the best ways to safeguard patients, and avoid legal headaches down the road.

Charting by exception: There are perils

A court's finding of negligence highlights the dangers of "charting by exception."

I f you're concerned about the legal risks of charting by exception, you have reason to be. At least one court—a United States court of appeals—has condemned the use of the practice in a case against a hospital in Puerto Rico. The decision suggests that charting by exception may be a perilous policy for other U.S. hospitals as well.

Charting by exception is defined as much by what is omitted from the patient's record as by what is included in it. Although the term means different things at different institutions and to different people, the general principle is to chart only when something unusual or out of the ordinary happens.

Some hospitals have adopted a policy of charting by exception, presumably in an effort to save time. And individual nurses may engage in this practice on their own, as a shortcut on a busy day. Either way, the court's decision should make administrators and nurses sit up and take notice, and perhaps reconsider.

A chart riddled with unanswered questions

On May 15, 1985, the patient, Roberto Romero Lama, underwent surgery for a herniated disk in a hospital in Puerto Rico. The first sign of a possible problem, judging from his chart, occurred on May 17, when a nurse noted that the bandage covering the surgical wound was "very bloody." An entry the next day indicates that the patient had pain at the incision site.

On May 19, the bandage appeared "soiled again," according to the chart. And on May 20, the record shows that the patient reported severe back pain. The next day a physician diagnosed diskitis, an infection in the space between disks, and ordered antibiotics.

A more complete picture of the patient's evolving condition isn't available because the hospital's policy called for nurses to chart by exception; they were to note qualitative observations only when necessary to chronicle important clinical changes. Although objective aspects of the patient's care and condition— such as temperature, vital signs, and medication administration—were charted regularly, important details like the changing characteristics of the surgical wound and the patient's reports of pain were not.

As a result, it's not clear what transpired between the time the nurse first documented the bloody bandage and when it was noted as soiled again, or between this time and when the patient developed severe pain. Were any nursing or medical interventions attempted, for example? Did the wound improve, or did there continue to be signs of a possible infection? Had the patient continued to report pain or any other symptoms to the nurses, and did the nurses consult with the patient's attending physician? Without answers to these questions, it is impossible to judge the care the patient received.

The jury did conclude—and the appeals court agreed—that more complete charting would have alerted doctors to the existence of an infection. And that would likely have led to earlier medical intervention, possibly preventing the diskitis and sparing the patient the several additional months of hospitalization needed to treat the infection. "Intermittent charting failed to provide the sort of continuous danger signals that would be the most likely to spur early intervention by a physician," the court of appeals noted in upholding the lower court's finding.[1]

Key to the court's finding was the fact that the hospital's charting policy violated a regulation of the Puerto Rico Department of Health, which requires qualitative nurses' notes for each nursing shift. The court upheld the jury's award for the plaintiff—$600,000 in compensatory damages.

The dangers of selective charting

The charting in this instance fell short by any standards—since even conditions that deviated from the patient's norm were not documented, as generally called for under a charting-by-exception policy.[2] Nonetheless, the case does highlight some dangers you need to be aware of.

The streamlined approach of charting by exception can make it difficult to prove the attentiveness of the nursing staff in the event a problem arises and a lawsuit results. More importantly, it could contribute to the condition that triggers a negligence claim in the first place—by not providing caregivers who review the chart with a thorough picture of the patient's evolving condition.

Because of these risks, it's very important that you pay strict attention to charting parameters—more than you would with copious amounts of record-keeping—if you work in a hospital that has a charting-by-exception policy. Begin by finding out exactly what is expected to be included in the patient's record. Good charting by exception includes the use of well-designed flow sheets—enabling nurses to note all normal findings with a simple check mark, for example.[2]

If you think that your hospital's charting policy is ambiguous or unsafe in some way, confer with other nurses and your supervisor and then approach an administrator about clarifying or improving it. Ask for a written policy on charting, if none exists. You may also want to suggest charting as a topic for periodic inservices for the nursing staff.

Consider, too, bringing the risks of a charting-by-exception policy—to both the hospital and the patient—to the attention of your facility's risk manager or legal counsel. Ask about compliance with state health department regulations for charting.

As a practical matter, of course, you can't chart everything, no matter what kind of policy you have. You have to use common sense and sound judgment. Still, any significant indicator of the patient's condition or a change in status should be charted, along with corresponding interventions and the patient's response. The chart must accurately reflect the patient's condition and progress; that may mean documenting certain observations in detail—the color, consistency, and quantity of drainage, for example. Significant deficits—such as lethargy or lack of response—should also be charted.

If a claim is filed that puts your record-keeping under scrutiny, you will be judged by the following standard: Would a reasonably prudent nurse of similar education, training, and experience have charted this way? If the answer is Yes, your defense will be on solid ground; if the answer is No, the damage to your credibility can undermine your hospital's defense.

Quite simply, good charting is worth its weight in gold. It means safer care for your patient, and a sounder defense for you and your hospital should a lawsuit arise.

REFERENCES

1. Lama v. Borras, 16 F.3d 473 PR (1st Cir.1994).
2. Yocum, F. (1993). Documentation Skills For Quality Patient Care. Tipp City, OH: Awareness Productions.

Policies and procedures: Protection or peril?

While most written policies offer legal backup to the nurses who follow them, some actually increase risk. Here's how you can tell the difference.

Ask most nurses about policies and protocols, and they'll tell you to follow them to the letter. Deviating from a written procedure, they say, can jeopardize patient safety and incur liability. Yet a recent case reveals another side of the picture: A jury's finding of nursing negligence may have had more to do with the wording of a policy than with the actions of the nurses.

To reap the protective benefits of an institutional protocol, the staff members affected by it would be wise to take a closer look—and then to press for modifications if necessary. When you are presented with a new or revised written policy, consider whether it accurately reflects your nursing practice, and whether it's realistic to expect you to follow it. Narrow parameters— declaring that post-operative cardiac patients need a tidal volume of 800 before extubation, for example—often make effective guidelines. But turning such parameters into require- ments can be a legal booby trap because there are bound to be patients for whom such levels cannot be reached.

Consider, too, whether you have received the training you need to fully understand and follow a new or revised procedure. And think about the various duties you perform. Is there an aspect of your job that's not covered by a policy, but should be because it's outside the usual scope of nursing practice? Even worse, is there a task that you're expected to perform that violates an existing policy? A review of some cases and problems will help you accurately assess the policies and protocols of your institution.

If a policy promises more than it delivers

"When a woman who is in labor arrives in L&D, nurses must examine her vaginally to determine the baby's position." So stated a policy for the OB unit of an Illinois hospital. At first glance, that seems reasonable. Yet a jury and an appeals court found negligence on the part of nurses who apparently did their best to follow it.

The problem began when the patient was admitted at about 1:00 a.m., with contractions eight minutes apart. The admitting nurse reviewed the woman's history and medical records, performed the required vaginal exam, and called the attending obstetrician to report that the baby was in a vertex position.

For the next five hours, nurses conducted periodic follow-up exams and kept in touch with the doctor, who eventually ordered pitocin (Oxytocin). When he came to the hospital to examine the patient and rupture the membranes, the doctor, like the nurses, found the baby in a vertex position.

For several more hours, labor and follow-up exams proved uneventful. Then, some 14 hours after the woman was admitted, a nurse's vaginal exam revealed that the cervix was fully dilated—but that the baby was breech.

The doctor, summoned at once, arrived in minutes, but too late to perform a cesarean. Delivered vaginally, the infant sustained permanent kidney damage from the obstetrician's attempted rotation. The parents sued, charging the doctor, nurses, and hospital with negligence.

There's nothing unusual about finding negligence when an infant is injured. What's unusual is that the nurses seem to have met the appropriate standard of care—performing and documenting regular exams, and keeping in close touch with the doctor. But, despite an expert's testimony that it's difficult to determine a baby's position before the membranes are ruptured or the cervix is 9 cm dilated, the jury and appeals court found that it wasn't enough: The RNs should have determined earlier that the baby was breech.

The wording of the hospital's policy—that nurses must determine the position—is the likely reason the staff reported conclusive rather than ambiguous findings. Thus, it set an unrealistic standard that even the most conscientious nurses could not meet. And while the court attributed most of the negligence to the obstetrician, the poorly written policy still cost the hospital well over half a million dollars for its portion of a massive $2.9 million award.

A clear-cut policy is worth its weight in gold

Fortunately, most written policies are unambiguous and fairly easy to follow. One of their major benefits is to lend support to nurses who find themselves in the uncomfortable position of having to go over an administrator's head or refuse to follow a physician's order.

The story of a patient who died suddenly, less than a day after PACU nurses refused to follow a doctor's order to administer nitroprusside (Nipride), is a case in point. Despite the unexpected death, no liability was attributed to the doctor, the nurses, or the hospital. The reason? Because nitroprusside requires continuous monitoring, hospital policy stated that the drug be administered only in the ICU.

Faced with the nurses' refusal, the doctor had administered another antihypertensive, then given nitroprusside—which the patient did not respond well to—after transferring the patient to the intensive care unit. But the court found neither the delay nor the nitroprusside responsible for the death. Had the nurses violated hospital policy and administered the nitroprusside in the PACU, though, the patient's poor response to the drug would likely have left them in a precarious legal position.

When to push for a policy, how to evaluate it

An OR nurse at a small hospital often holds the retractors during surgical procedures, a task performed by surgical residents at most larger facilities. What should she do?

A nurse anesthetist contracts with a hospital whose policy calls for her to work only under the direct supervision of an anesthesiologist. Yet there are occasions when the supervising physician wanders out into the lounge or supervises several other CRNAs simultaneously. What should this nurse do?

Both nurses worry, justifiably, about liability. Their job, and yours any time you're faced with a task or responsibility that conflicts with hospital policy or that may be outside the ordinary scope of nursing practice, is to discuss the problem with the department supervisor at once. Follow up with your hospital risk manager.

If the work you're doing, like that of the nurse who holds the retractors, is highly unusual, verify that it's within the scope of your state's nurse practice act. If a policy is too broad, press for specifics—such as an explanation of just what "direct supervision" involves. When a policy is not or cannot be adhered to, notify your supervisor, in writing.

Use these guidelines whenever you evaluate a written policy, whether it's a new one or one that's being revised or updated:

- The policy should be neither too broad nor too narrow. It should establish standards that can be met.
- Staff members who will be affected by a policy should be involved in writing or revising it.
- Policies should be reviewed periodically, preferably once a year, and outdated protocols revised to reflect current practice.

- Inservices on all new or rewritten policies and procedures should always be provided, with attendance mandatory and documented.
- Once staff members receive training in a particular protocol, they should be held responsible for following it.
- Copies of all applicable policies and protocols should be easily accessible, so they can be consulted as needed.[1,2]

The reward for your diligence? Policies that protect rather than imperil.

REFERENCES

1. Staff. (1992, Aug./Sept.). Don't set standards that can't be met. Patient Care Law, 3.

2. Calloway, S. D., & Kota, J. M. (1989). Legal issues in supervising nurses (2nd ed.). Eau Claire, WI: Professional Education System.

Your role in informed consent

This update will help you distinguish between your responsibility and the physician's.

Consider this scenario: An Hispanic woman arrives on your unit the night before she's scheduled for a hysterectomy, clutching an unsigned consent form. You call her doctor, who tells you she's been fully informed and asks you to obtain and witness her signature. There's just one problem: The consent form is written in English. The patient, Maria Ramos, has difficulty understanding and speaking the language.

Should you obtain the signature anyway, accepting the physician's assurance that Mrs. Ramos has been fully informed? Are you obligated to convey the risks and alternatives first? What does it mean to witness a patient's signature? And is it in fact your responsibility?

If you're not sure about the answers to these questions, you're not alone. For many nurses, the informed consent process is fraught with confusion. This review will clarify your role.

Providing information: When and how much?

Informed consent is a two-part process: giving the patient sufficient information so that she can make an educated choice, and getting her assent in writing. But when is informed consent needed? And how much information is enough?

For basic care such as bathing or taking vital signs, consent is implied by the patient's cooperation and presence in a hospital, office, or clinic. Hospital patients sign a general consent upon admission that covers routine diagnostics like X-rays and lab work. Procedures that could cause serious complications, however, require informed consent—a written explanation, accompanied by an oral description that includes alternatives and risks, which the patient must understand and sign to indicate assent. In life-threatening emergencies, of course, the consent process is waived.

Along with surgery, anesthesia, cardiac catheterizations, and other invasive procedures, tests with potentially sensitive out-comes—the blood test for HIV antibodies, for instance—usually require informed consent. For any experimental therapy, federal law mandates an even more stringent consent process.

Although courts have not ruled on precisely what information a patient should receive, it must include the nature and purpose of the procedure, the alternatives, and the risks. The explanation must be given in easily understood terms, not in medical jargon. It need not detail every minor complication. But it must cover any possible consequence severe enough to affect mental or physical functioning, and include facts that any reasonably prudent patient would need to make an intelligent decision about treatment.

Who conveys alternatives and risks?

The practitioner who orders or performs the procedure is held responsible for informing the patient about it. In traditional hospital settings, that's almost always the physician. Discussing the risks of and alternatives to a hysterectomy with Maria Ramos is not her nurse's duty.

That is not to say that the duty to inform belongs exclusively to physicians. In three separate decisions—each of them involving nurses administering immunizations in an outpatient setting—courts placed it squarely on nurses' shoulders. Each court ruled that because the nurses acted independently in assessing and weighing risks and benefits before deciding whether to administer the vaccine, they—not the doctors—bore the responsibility for informed consent.

As nurses gain increasing autonomy, particularly in their work outside the hospital, decisions like these are increasingly likely. In home care, for instance, nurses often rely on standing orders or protocols that require them to make the ultimate decision on whether to give a drug. In doing so, one legal analyst points out, the nurse becomes the "learned intermediary," and incurs the duty to alert patients to alternatives and risks.[1]

Legally, a nurse with a reasonable belief that a patient has been adequately informed by the physician can ask for and witness his signature. Although it's recommended—and increasingly likely— that hospitals require doctors to do this themselves, many nurses will take part in the process. Your hospital should have a written policy defining the role of nursing staff. If it doesn't, talk to your supervisor or risk manager about developing one.

A nurse as witness: What does it mean?

When you sign a consent form as a witness, your signature attests to three things: authenticity, capacity, and voluntariness. Authenticity means you attest to the fact that the signature obtained is the patient's. But a signature alone is meaningless unless the patient understands what it is he's signed. As the witness, you must have reason to believe that the patient has the capacity for understanding—that he was verbally apprised of the nature of the procedure and alternatives and risks, read the form, understands it, and agrees to submit to the proposed treatment. Finally, your signature indicates that the patient signed without force or coercion.

If you were present while the doctor talked to the patient and if you heard the patient's response, being a witness is likely to be easy. If you were not, ask if the doctor talked to him about the procedure and then allowed him to ask questions. Assuming that the answer is Yes, have the patient read the form carefully and assure you that he understands it. Watch while he signs it. If a language barrier or other communication problem prevents you from confirming that the patient was properly informed, refuse to act as the witness.

Do not allow a patient to sign the form, either, if he says he doesn't understand or has not been fully informed, or if he seems unsure. Instead, notify the doctor at once. The procedure must not proceed until all of the patient's questions have been answered.

When circumstances change the rules

When a patient is a minor, does not speak the language, or is unable to read or write, it complicates the informed consent process. In most states, children under 18 lack the capacity to consent to medical treatment, although many states make exceptions for reproductive health, mental health, and substance abuse treatment.

To obtain the consent of a parent or legal guardian, remember these basic guidelines: In the case of divorce, seek the consent of the custodial parent. Adoptive parents can give consent; stepparents cannot. The authority of foster parents varies from state to state. Unless you have reason to suspect legal problems, a simple question about an adult's relationship to the child will do.

When a child needs prompt treatment but no parent is present, telephone consent is the best substitute. Most hospitals require the doctor and a nurse or other witness to be on the line together. The physician explains the child's condition and the proposed treatment, complications, alternatives, and risks, while the nurse witnesses the explanation and the consent.

If a patient can understand what's on a consent form but can't read it because of illiteracy, visual impairment, or a language barrier, you or an interpreter should read the consent form aloud to her verbatim. Ask the patient if she understands what's been read and what she's being asked to sign. Obtain the signature only if the patient says Yes. If an interpreter is unavailable, notify your supervisor and the attending physician at once. Explain that you can't proceed because you're unable to attest to the patient's understanding.

If a patient cannot sign the form, because of paralysis or trauma, for instance, have her designate someone else to sign. To witness such a consent, observe the patient's verbal consent and the appointment and signature of the designee, who signs his own name and adds, "for Susan Jones." An illiterate patient can indicate consent with an X.

Documentation: The final step

No matter where you fit into the informed consent process, your documentation is crucial. The individual who provides information about the procedure documents that the discussion took place and what was discussed. If you serve as witness, protect yourself by charting the fact that you heard the doctor and patient discuss the procedure or that the patient told you the doctor had informed him fully.

Whenever a third party is involved—a guardian, interpreter, or designate—note his name and relationship to the patient. If you witness a telephone consent, chart the reason it was needed and the information conveyed.

Finally, keep in mind that a patient who consents to a procedure can change his mind. If a patient tells you he is unwilling to go forward at any step of the way, notify the doctor immediately to assure that the procedure does not take place. In such cases, or when a patient revokes his consent and then changes his mind again, thorough documentation is especially crucial.

Depending on circumstances, informed consent can be simple or complicated. Either way, your primary objective is to protect your patients.

REFERENCES

1. Tyler, J.S. (1991). The nurse as the learned intermediary: A new twist to an old rule. Drug Product Liability Reporter, 4(7), 98.

Reducing the risks of phone triage

Telephone triage has become an integral part of nursing practice. Learn how to handle the legal risks that come with the territory.

"My uncle just collapsed and is clutching his chest." "I had surgery last week and today my incision looks redder than it did a few days ago." "I want to die and I'm going to take a bottle of pills." "I'm pregnant and my back is killing me. What should I do?"

Nurses in all settings—hospitals, clinics, physicians' offices, and HMOs—are hearing questions, concerns, and pleas for help like these. Not from patients they can reach out and touch, but from callers on the other end of a telephone line.

With no visual clues to rely on and often no patient history to refer to, nurses who handle these calls often worry about the risks of "nursing by phone." If you answer calls from patients, here's what you need to know to minimize the legal risks for you and your employer.

Heed the advice of nursing groups

As far as calls to the emergency department go, the Emergency Nurses Association (ENA) has taken the position that, in the best interest of the patient, nurses should refrain from giving advice over the phone. Emergency situations, where instructions are necessary to prevent loss of life or limb, are the exception.[1]

Unless that's the case, the ENA recommends that nurses inform callers that their condition cannot be diagnosed over the phone and that they should either come to the ED or go to their personal physician for a complete evaluation.[1]

The ENA does, however, recognize that telephone triage programs do exist, and the need for them to be based on clearly defined protocols. Similarly, many state nursing boards have emphasized that assessment and evaluation over the telephone be performed only with specific protocols or standing orders.

Most nursing boards also agree that giving nursing advice over the telephone requires independent judgment and skill, and therefore cannot be delegated to LPNs, unlicensed personnel, or an office receptionist.[2,3] These staff members should collect only basic information such as the patient's name, telephone number, and chief complaint, and then put the call through to an RN or physician.

Work only with written guidelines

Symptom-based telephone protocols and standing orders—for purposes of this discussion, we'll refer to them both as protocols—offer a number of advantages: They help protect you from charges of practicing medicine without a license. They promote consistent treatment between patients with similar symptoms. And, if litigation arises years later, they can be used to reconstruct what advice was given—and, therefore, whether the standard of care was met.

Protocols also help ensure more accurate assessments by helping you to elicit the right information from callers. Studies of telephone triage calls have shown that inadequate history-taking is a common problem.[4]

Take, for example, the triage nurse who received a call from a mother whose 5-year-old daughter had been stung by a bee. After determining that the child did not show signs of an allergic reaction, the nurse advised the mother to apply ice and meat tenderizer to the wound. What the nurse failed to do was ask about the location of the sting—which turned out to be on the child's eyelid. Two days later, the child arrived at the ED with symptoms of acute chemical conjunctivitis and possible blindness.[5]

Had this nurse been using a telephone protocol, she would have been reminded of what questions to ask—in this case, the location of the wound. In a well-developed protocol, the questions—along with the corresponding nursing advice—are listed in descending order of importance. Those aimed at identifying the most emergent problems—like anaphylaxis in the case of the bee sting—come first.[4]

Symptoms for a particular complaint are categorized according to urgency as well. In that way, the protocol makes clear which patients need to be seen immediately, which can be seen by a physician the next day, and which can be given instructions for care at home.

If you're working with a protocol that doesn't address a particular symptom that your patient has, or if you feel the need to deviate from the protocol in any way, contact the physician before proceeding. If the physician is not available, tell the caller to go to the ED or come in to the office.

Protocols may be part of a published reference guide approved by the medical staff or a specific attending physician. Or, they can be specifically written by the medical staff for your particular patient population and facility.

Whichever sort of protocol you use, be sure there's a master copy, signed by the appropriate physician, on file. Make sure, too, that the protocols are reviewed regularly to ensure that they are consistent with current standards of care.

Be specific about the need to follow your advice

Once you've assessed the caller's problem and given the appropriate instructions, you need to try to ensure patient compliance. You don't want him claiming later that he didn't understand the urgency of his condition and the consequences of ignoring your advice.

Consider the case of the 16-year-old who dove into a pool and hit the bottom. A family member called the ED when the teen complained of neck pain, numbness, and a tingling in his arms

and legs. The triage nurse told the caller not to move the teen
and to call 911 at once. Instead, the patient arrived at the ED
three hours later, sitting up in the back seat of a car.[5]

In a case like this, where you're dealing with a possible
medical emergency, obtain the caller's address and keep him on
the line while either you or a colleague call 911. Stay on the line
until emergency medical technicians arrive.

If the condition is less urgent, state your instructions clearly
and give a specific time frame in which to seek medical attention
in person. It's not enough to tell the caller to go to the ED. Say,
"I recommend that you come to the ED within the next hour
because your situation seems urgent. What do you plan to do?"[5]

To convey the urgency of the situation, you may need to give a
working diagnosis. Choose your words carefully to avoid giving an
actual medical diagnosis. You might, for instance, tell a patient
that his symptoms suggest that he may have an injury to his spine.

Ward off liability through documentation

If a caller sues you claiming that you gave him improper advice,
a complete record of your conversation can save you from liability.
At the very least, document the date and time of the call, the
nature of the problem—quoting the patient, whenever possible—and the advice you gave. If you deviated from a protocol,
be sure to record your reasons, your discussion with the physician,
and any actions you took under the physician's direction.

Note the caller's name and phone number, too. Sometimes,
however, this won't be possible or prudent: If the caller is
threatening suicide, for example, you may need to spend time
gaining his trust rather than collecting data. On the other hand,
if he hangs up without giving you his name or phone number,
you've lost all chance of intervention.[4] There's nothing more
you can do except document the conversation, using quotes
whenever possible.

If the situation allows, record the patient's age and medical history including recent injuries, illnesses, and infections, allergies, and current medications. Be sure to record both positive and negative responses to your inquiries.

To document these calls, use standardized forms such as an encounter form—on which data from each call is recorded on a separate form—or a telephone log sheet—on which 25 to 30 calls are recorded on one page. Don't forget to sign your name after any notes you make. You can use your initials, as long as a legend with your initials and signature is included on each page of the form.

Encounter forms and telephone logs are not considered a part of a patient's medical record in all states, so there may be no legal requirement to retain them. To be on the safe side, though, operate as if there is a legal requirement to keep them: Maintain encounter forms of calls from former or current patients in the outpatient progress notes or on a 5 ½" x 8 ½" sheet of paper that you include in the medical record. Keep a separate file, arranged chronologically, for telephone logs.

Following appropriate protocols, promoting compliance, and documenting the advice you give over the phone will ensure the most appropriate care for the patient and the best legal protection for you and your employer.

REFERENCES

1. Emergency Nurses Association. (1996). Emergency Nurses Association position: Telephone advice. Park Ridge, IL: Author.
2. Wisconsin Board of Nursing. (1990). Telephone triage. Wisconsin Regulatory Digest, 3(2), 2.
3. National Council of State Boards of Nursing. (1994). Burbach v. Delegation in nursing. Issues, 15(3), 7.
4. Wheeler, S. Q., & Windt, J. H. (1993). Telephone triage: Theory, practice, and protocol development. Albany, NY: Delmar Publishers.
5. Wheeler, S. Q. (1989). ED telephone triage: Lessons learned from unusual calls. J. Emerg. Nurs., 15(6), 481.

When communication breaks down

Failing to communicate with clinicians or patients can have dire consequences for all concerned. Do you know the ground rules you should be following?

The importance of communicating key information to colleagues and patients seems obvious. So why are foul-ups in communication the basis for so many malpractice claims?

There are several reasons. Some nurses assume that the patient's doctor is already aware of the information. Others are reluctant to bother the physician. Nurses who are working in offices or clinics may not know how far they should go in relaying information to patients. And nurses in any setting may not realize their obligation to track down information—such as lab work or radiology reports—from those who've neglected to provide it.

The reason for the communication breakdown won't matter much to a jury if a patient comes to harm as a result, as the cases presented here make clear. Knowing the guidelines for communicating information or retrieving it from others will help you safeguard your patients and minimize your risk of liability.

What you need to tell physicians

The standard of care requires you to inform the treating physician about anything significant that the patient or family member has told you or that you yourself have observed. In a recent Georgia case, the plaintiff claimed that a triage nurse's failure to relay certain facts to a physician was partly responsible for a baby's lifelong disability.[1]

The mother of the baby boy, who'd been diagnosed with a respiratory infection not long before, called the after-hours phone line of her managed care plan. She told the nurse that her child had a fever of 104° and was panting, moaning, and limp. The nurse directed the mother to place the baby in a cool bath while she contacted the on-call pediatrician.

The nurse told the pediatrician that she had ruled out respiratory distress, but did not report the baby's symptoms of panting and moaning. The pediatrician did not consider the baby's condition critical, and instructed the nurse to tell the mother to take the baby to a children's medical center that was 40 miles from the mother's home.

En route, the baby went into respiratory and cardiac arrest. He was resuscitated at a nearby hospital, but color never returned to his extremities. Gangrene soon developed, and the baby's hands and part of each leg had to be amputated.

The child was diagnosed with meningococcemia, a rare blood infection that can necessitate amputation. But the baby's family sued the managed care plan, claiming that negligence on the part of the nurse and physician had delayed treatment that could have prevented the gangrene. They were awarded $45 million by a jury.

Failing to relay specific symptoms—in this case the panting and moaning—is always risky, but particularly so if the nurse is in the role of gatekeeper, as is the case with many HMOs, clinics, and private practices. In such instances, the physician must often depend solely on the nurse's interpretation of the information to make his own medical judgment. So, whenever possible, relay to the doctor the exact words the caller used to describe the symptoms.

When you're caring for a patient in person, you're in a better position to assess symptoms and their significance. But certain information still needs to be communicated directly to the physician, not just charted. There's no golden rule for determining exactly what information should be communicated—you'll have to ask yourself how critical the facts are to the patient's diagnosis and treatment and then make a nursing judgment.

Keep in mind that merely communicating the information isn't enough; how swiftly you do so also counts. The time frame should be commensurate with the significance of the information. Unfortunately, many nurses are reluctant to bother physicians and prefer to wait until the doctor comes to the hospital for rounds. That may prove to be too late.

If you're unsure whether the information you have warrants contacting the doctor, discuss the matter with a colleague or your nursing supervisor. If your findings demand immediate attention and the doctor is unreachable, give the information to the person who's next in your hospital's chain of command.

A general word of warning: Never assume that the doctor or other members of the health care team are aware of all key facts, especially if you notice actions that don't correspond with what you know about the patient. Be alert to any discrepancies between your assessment and the doctor's interventions, and question them.

Back up your actions with solid charting

Once you transmit information to the physician, be sure to document that you have done so. It's not unusual for cases of botched communication to boil down to the word of the doctor against the word of the nurse. Here's an example:

A nurse examined a woman who had come to the hospital in labor and found the baby in breech position. According to the nurse, she called the woman's doctor and told him about the breech presentation. The doctor told her he would wait a while before coming to the hospital unless he was urgently needed. After hanging up the phone, the nurse spoke with a colleague and telephoned the doctor back to tell him that the situation was indeed critical and he should come in right away.[2]

The doctor claimed that he was called only once, was told the presentation was indeterminate, and that, nonetheless, he immediately left for the hospital. He said if he had been told of the breech, he would have instructed the nurse to prepare for an emergency caesarean section so surgery could be done as soon as he arrived.

As it turned out, surgery was delayed because no preparations had been made and the hospital had only antiquated equipment on hand. With birth imminent the baby was delivered vaginally, resulting in complications that left the baby with a physical disability. The family sued the obstetrician, anesthesiologist, and community hospital, eventually settling for $435,000.

Had the case been tried, the nurse would have been in a position to defend herself against the obstetrician's word, because her nursing notes supported her version of events. In a case of "he said, she said," documentation is a nurse's best ally. But pay attention to how you document.

Be sure to always write the date and time of your entry next to your notes; specify when the actual event took place within the note. Document all attempts to reach the doctor, and make clear who is doing the calling. For instance, if you phoned the doctor and simply charted your actions as "M.D. called" it can be interpreted as meaning that the physician phoned you.

Similarly, writing "Discussed symptoms with Dr. Smith," leaves the reader unclear as to whether you imparted information to the physician or he to you. Instead, you should write "I called Dr. Smith and advised him of the following ..." Document the physician's response, and the source of the information you conveyed—whether your own observations, reports from a patient or relative, or word from a lab.

When someone neglects to communicate with you

It's not just doctors you need to communicate closely with, but labs and clinical departments that process test results, as well. While such communication is a two-way street, it may be incumbent on you to clear away any roadblocks. Here's a case in point:

A woman went to a Texas hospital complaining of a spider bite. She had an elevated white count and an ongoing infection, and was suspected of having diabetes. Blood work was ordered and sent to an outside lab. The results indicated an extremely high glucose level.[3]

The lab knew the results late that afternoon and transmitted them to the hospital a few hours later by teletype. However, neither the patient's nurses nor the treating physician looked at the results until the next morning. By that time the patient had slipped into a ketoacidotic coma. She died soon after.

The lab's policies and procedures required technicians to call the hospital with results of panic values. A lab tech claimed he had done that, but could not identify who he had spoken with. Nurses hadn't made a point of checking the teletype machine because it was supposed to contain only routine lab results. The woman's estate sued the hospital, two nurses, the lab, and the doctor, and eventually settled for a total of $455,000.

Whenever tests are ordered, it's your responsibility to check for results in a reasonable period of time; if they haven't been received, it's up to you to call the lab to find out why.

The same sort of follow-up is indicated with tests or referrals ordered in an office or outpatient setting. Every office or clinic should have a system to track consultations, lab work, radiology reports, and the like. If a report isn't received, a nurse should call the appropriate office to find out why and document that she has done so. If the patient never went for the test in the first place, you may need to follow up directly with him.

Your duty to patients

If you work in an office, clinic, or ED, how far should you go to communicate information—such as suspicious test results or misread X-rays—to patients who don't respond to an initial phone call?

Just how long or diligently you try to contact the patient depends on how potentially serious the test results are. If the findings suggest or confirm a condition that requires further treatment, you need to follow up your call with a letter—return receipt requested—and repeat calls. The letter should explicitly state what the finding is and its significance, and the need for further evaluation or treatment.

Be sure to document each of your attempts to contact the patient, including the date and time of the call and the end result—line busy, no answer, left message on answering machine, whatever. If you do reach the patient, document the substance of your conversation. Also, keep a copy of all letters that are sent in the patient's chart.

When leaving messages for patients at their home or office, be discreet. Communicating information to the wrong person— the results of a pregnancy test to a teenager's parent, for example—can cause serious problems for the patient and expose you to a breach of confidentiality claim. So can communicating information in the wrong manner—leaving the results of an HIV test on an answering machine, for example.

If you have to leave a message on a machine say something like "This is Nurse Michaels from Dr. Frederick's office. Please call the office as soon as possible." Don't say anything about diagnosis, prognosis, or treatment.

Prudence should always guide your communications. That, and a willingness to err on the side of caution when speaking directly with patients or members of the health care team: Better too much communication than not enough.

REFERENCES

1. $45,000,000 verdict, negligent failure to follow proper protocol over the telephone in determining whether emergency medical care was necessary. (July 1995). Medical Litigation Alert, 3(11), 16.

2. A $435,000 settlement for an Erb's palsy. (1994). Professional Liability Newsletter, 24(12), 3.

3. Medical Malpractice Verdicts, Settlements & Experts. (1994). 10(12), 24.

Protecting patients' privacy

Confidentiality rules can be tricky to follow. But understanding them and taking steps to avoid breaches can keep you out of legal trouble.

P rotecting the confidentiality of a patient's health information used to be as simple as securing his chart from unauthorized eyes and holding discussions with or about him out of earshot of those who did not provide direct patient care.

Today, it's much more problematic. State laws and court rulings have created a number of exceptions to general confidentiality requirements. Public concern over sensitive issues such as HIV and genetic test results has led to a debate about special protections to ensure patients' privacy. And technology has increased the ways patient information can be shared and, therefore, the number of people who have access to it.

Every nurse, then, needs to know when and how to protect a patient's right to privacy—a right based on the U.S. Constitution and upheld by laws in all 50 states. Here's a look at the key issues and liability risks.

When are you compelled to disclose?

You have a legal duty to report certain situations in which the safety of the patient or the welfare of the public is considered at risk. Most jurisdictions require reporting of child and elder abuse and other illegal actions, situations in which the patient may harm another, and communicable diseases. Because reporting requirements vary by state, you'll need to check with your risk manager or local statutes for specific provisions in your jurisdiction.

In general, however, as long as you report in good faith and according to the law, most statutes provide immunity from civil and criminal liability. And failure to report could subject you to a fine and disciplinary action.

Here are the four main exceptions to the rule of patient-provider confidentiality:

Child and elder abuse. Every state requires nurses and physicians to report cases of suspected child abuse, neglect, and abandonment to the appropriate state agency or the police. A child is generally defined as anyone under the age of 18.

All states also require nurses in nursing homes to report cases of suspected elder abuse, neglect, and abandonment. Most states impose the same reporting requirement on nurses in other settings as well. The definition of an elderly patient varies—in Connecticut, for example, it's anyone over the age of 60—and some statutes don't specify an age.

Follow your employer's reporting policy. Document all observations of suspected abuse or neglect in the patient's chart, both physical (bruises, lesions, and so on) and psychological (fear or a withdrawn disposition).

Other criminal activity. All 50 states mandate that rape cases be reported to the police.[1] In some jurisdictions, narcotic use or evidence of violent crimes—such as gunshot or stab wounds—must be reported, as well.

Recently, Illinois and Oregon enacted laws that weaken the confidentiality rights of patients being treated for motor vehicle accident injuries. These states now allow health care providers to notify police about the results of blood or urine tests that show alcohol or drug levels above the legal limit. Maine has a similar law. It states that if an RN or other provider knows or reasonably suspects that a patient who has been involved in a motor vehicle accident has been driving while under the influence of alcohol or drugs, she may report this to the police. So, nurses in these states who wish to report drivers who are drunk or high can do so without legal repercussions.

Dangerous patients. If a patient tells you that he is going to harm another person, you may be obligated to disclose that information to protect the intended victim. That duty was established more than 20 years ago with the landmark Tarasoff case, in which the California Supreme Court found a psychotherapist liable for failing to warn a woman of his patient's plan to kill her—a plan that was carried out.[2]

If your patient makes such a threat, document it in his chart—in quotes and in his exact words, if possible—and question him further. If you believe the threat has merit, immediately inform your supervisor, risk manager, or the physician so that appropriate actions can be taken to avert harm.

Communicable diseases. Certain infectious conditions must be reported to the appropriate state or local agency or health department. The most controversial disease on the reporting list: HIV/AIDS.

Every state requires the reporting of AIDS cases for epidemiological purposes—some require the reporting of the patient's name and address, while others prohibit the disclosure of any identifying data. Moreover, 28 states mandate the reporting—by name—of patients diagnosed with HIV. Some states also permit disclosure of a patient's HIV-positive status to third parties—say, a sexual partner or needle-sharing partner. However, many states allow only a physician or a public health officer—not the patient's nurse—to disclose this information.

When disclosure requires consent

Generally, informational data such as a patient's name, address, and dates of admission or discharge are not considered confidential information and therefore not protected by law. Information related to diagnosis, treatment, and prognosis, however, is considered confidential. Before disclosing this information to anyone other than members of the health care team—and unless otherwise mandated by law or a court order—obtain your patient's consent.

Verbal consent, either implicit or explicit, is usually sufficient to discuss your patient's health face-to-face with concerned relatives or friends. Try to avoid disclosing such information over the phone, whenever possible. You never know who is really on the other end of the line.

But for anyone else—and especially when sending his actual medical records—obtain written authorization from the patient or, if he's unconscious, his representative.

In most cases, this can simply be a signed letter from the patient or a signed, general consent form, such as the kind insurance companies use. In certain instances, however, a general letter or release is not enough.

Information related to a patient's HIV/AIDS status (other than that governed by the disclosure rules discussed earlier), psychiatric condition, and drug or alcohol treatment receives special protection from disclosure under federal and state laws. You are prohibited from releasing any such information—including the patient's name or dates of admission or discharge—without your patient's specific consent.

As with a general release form, a patient's specific consent must be in writing, dated, and signed by him or his proxy. It must also state the purpose of the disclosure, the specific data to be revealed, to whom it can be revealed, who can make the disclosure, and how long the consent is valid.

When sending specially protected health information through the mail, make sure that it's accompanied by a statement of confidentiality, which prohibits the receiving party from revealing the information without the patient's consent. If you're disclosing the information verbally, you're not dutybound to recite this statement—but it certainly wouldn't hurt.

Currently, no special cloak of protection exists for another sensitive type of health information—genetic test results. But that could change as more and more patients are tested for genes that mutate to cancer and other diseases.

Genetic information has raised fears by patients that employers will discriminate against them and that insurance companies will deny or limit coverage. Some women who carry genes linked to breast or ovarian cancer are asking their doctors not to include this information in their medical records. Some doctors are complying with these requests, relying instead on their memories and pretending not to know any genetic information when dealing with insurers and other physicians.[3]

It's a thorny issue—what to do if a patient asks you not to chart potentially explosive information pertaining to diagnosis, prognosis, or treatment. At this point, it remains largely an ethical call that each health care professional must make for him- or herself.

Technology brings legal pitfalls, too

Developments in communication technology have made the business of caring for patients more efficient. But using computers, fax machines, videotapes, and telephones to process, store, or transmit patient information has set the stage for security violations like never before.

Fortunately, the federal government has stepped in to help. The Health Insurance Portability and Accountability Act of 1996 mandates, among other things, that Congress establish privacy rules to manage electronic records within three and a half years of the law's enactment. These rules must stipulate that anyone with access to computerized health information be given training on maintaining confidentiality.

You should, however, already be taking steps to ensure the privacy of electronic information. If you use a computer by the patient's bedside or at the nurse's station, clear the screen after each use. Position the screen in a way that passersby cannot see it. And, don't give your password to anyone.

Keep videotapes and backup computer disks—as well as paper records—in a secure place for the amount of time required by law. Never reuse tapes or disks because they may not be completely erased.

Avoid faxing medical information whenever possible. If it's unavoidable, verify the number you'll be sending the fax to and determine in advance that an authorized party will be on hand to receive it as soon as it comes in.

When providing health information over the phone, do so in a private area. Always verify to whom you are speaking and whether that person is entitled to information about a patient's health. If the party you are calling is not in, don't leave a message that reveals anything about a patient's condition. Instead ask to have the party you are trying to reach return the call.

Of course, many breaches of confidentiality have nothing to do with technology at all. They occur when providers discuss confidential data in areas where they can be overheard. Hold all such discussions in a private location, away from unauthorized ears. When talking to a patient who is not in a private room, remember to keep your voice down.

Trust is a cornerstone of the patient-provider relationship. Making sure your patient's health information stays confidential will help you uphold that trust. Understanding the exceptions to confidentiality rules in select situations will help put you on a course that's liability-free.

REFERENCES

1. Greve, P. A. (1990). Keep quiet or speak up? Issues in patient confidentiality. RN, 53(12), 53.
2. Tarasoff v. The Regents of the University of California, 13 Cal. 3d 177, 529 P.2d 553 (1974).
3. Kolata, G. (1997, February 4). Advent of testing for breast cancer genes leads to fears of disclosure and discrimination. The New York Times, p. C1.

Implications of the Patient Self-Determination Act

Informing patients
about end-of-life treatment choices,
determining their wishes—
and respecting them—can be difficult.
You can help.

I t's supposed to work this way: An elderly stroke victim, hemiplegic and aphasic, is wheeled onto your med/surg unit. You see in his medical record that he has prepared an advance directive; a copy of his living will is attached. A week later, after suffering a second stroke, the man becomes comatose. Following his documented wishes, caregivers agree to withhold CPR and other life support measures, and the patient dies peacefully in his sleep—the way he wanted to.

In the real world, you are just as likely to face this situation: The patient arrives on your unit barely conscious and in critical condition. By the time you have a free moment to ask about an advance directive, he's unable to answer, so you approach his distraught wife. On the verge of tears, all she can tell you is, "I know he has a living will, but I don't know where it is."

You document this in his medical record and inform the doctor. But when the patient arrests later that night, the code team revives him—and then hooks him up to a ventilator, over his wife's objections. When the attending physician later asks the patient's wife if she would like to have it stopped, she says No, unwilling to take the responsibility for what she refers to as "pulling the plug." The patient remains on the ventilator in a coma for two more weeks until he dies, without ever regaining consciousness.

Encouraging living wills and health care proxies

The Patient Self-Determination Act (PSDA), which took effect in December 1991, was intended to make it easier for individuals to express their preferences about medical treatment, particularly about terminal care, and easier for health care providers to honor those preferences. The law requires all federally funded hospitals to inform adult patients, in writing, about their right, under state law, to make treatment choices, including Do Not Resuscitate (DNR) orders.

The PSDA stipulates that patients must be asked if they have prepared a living will or executed a durable power of attorney for health care, which allows a proxy to make medical decisions if the patient becomes incompetent. Currently, all states either have living will laws or recognize such documents as evidence of a patient's wishes.

What the PSDA does not stipulate is how hospitals can comply with the law, or which department or group of caregivers should be involved in implementing it. Because nurses spend so much time with patients and have opportunities to talk about advance directives, they often play a key role: Nurses can help overcome the problems that still limit exercise of this patient right to make terminal and other care choices.

The PSDA isn't a panacea. For one thing, most people still don't get around to preparing advance directives. So when they're admitted to a hospital, there is no written document to guide health care providers. Even patients who have signed a special medical directive rarely manage to bring it with them or have a loved one do so.

For another, nurses and other caregivers are frequently required to bring up the subject of advance directives at the worst possible time: at admission. Many patients are psychologically ill-prepared to confront such a basic question at this point, and some may become anxious or uncommunicative at the first mention of life support or living wills.

If a patient who hasn't prepared an advance directive is unconscious or cognitively impaired, treatment decisions may fall to his spouse, children, or other close relatives. They'll have advice from physicians, nurses, a chaplain, social worker, or members of the hospital's ethics committee; but, under great emotional strain, they may not be in a good position to make such life-or-death choices unless the matter has already been discussed. Too often, it hasn't. Out of ignorance, guilt, or denial, relatives sometimes demand that everything be done to keep a patient alive—which may not be what he would have wanted.

Why patients' wishes aren't always respected

Even when a patient has gone to great lengths to draw up a valid advance directive specifying the kind of life-sustaining treatment he wants and does not want—and even when a nurse attaches the document to his medical record and alerts the doctor—his wishes may not be carried out.

Why? First of all, the advance directive may never take effect: The conditions for honoring a living will or durable power of attorney may not be met. Depending on state law, living wills may only apply to patients diagnosed as terminally ill, or—under most state laws—in an irreversible condition such as a persistent vegetative state. While a durable power of attorney doesn't depend on terminal illness, it takes effect only when a patient loses the ability—even temporarily—to make decisions himself. As long as a patient can make rational decisions, caregivers should be guided by his expressed wishes. But sometimes, it's hard to say when that line is crossed.

What's more, health care providers don't always feel bound to honor living wills. They may believe the patient's wishes are ambiguous or that he had no way of anticipating specific treatment choices. They may object for medical reasons.

In fact, despite laws recognizing a patient's right to decide his fate, many states also provide immunity from suit for doctors who make good faith decisions about sustaining life—for example, if a patient is started on life support before the attending physician can review an advance directive. Nor do doctors face any major legal penalties if they disregard a patient's terminal care preferences. On the other hand, caregivers do worry about being sued if they follow a patient's documented wishes and ignore a family's insistence on "heroic" measures to keep him alive.

Then there's hospital policy. In some facilities, staff are trained to handle and encourage advance directives; in others, they are not. While most hospitals have gone beyond the letter of the PSDA—by sponsoring seminars on advance directives, for example—in some hospitals the PSDA is paid only lip service.

For example, a cardiac patient in Connecticut was admitted to three different hospitals, for two unsuccessful angioplasties and then bypass surgery. Only at the first, where he came in on a non-emergency basis, was he given any information about advance directives: An ill-at-ease admissions staffer handed him a packet of papers, saying "Look this over. It's up to you. We're required by law to give you this," and let it go at that. Entering through the ED at the other two hospitals, he wasn't asked or told anything about special medical directives.

Finally, there is the way paperwork is handled in a hospital. A patient may be admitted with a valid advance directive, and a copy may be attached to her medical record, but when she's transferred to another unit the document may not travel with her.

In this sensitive and complex matter, what is your appropriate role? Nurses often find themselves caught between attending physicians on the one hand and patients and their families on the other. How well conflicts get resolved can depend on how easy it is for the concerned parties to discuss advance directives—so that they can understand the options and the implications of their decisions.

You can help make tough choices easier

Be sure to talk to patients and their families about their right to refuse or accept medical treatment, even if you know they've already been told. You may be the only caregiver aware of the struggle over treatment decisions that a patient and her family are facing. If a patient expresses preferences, see that she has the opportunity to put her wishes in writing by executing an advance directive, and that it's noted in the medical record, communicated to other clinicians, kept with the patient, and respected. If a patient has already executed an advance directive, but it's at home, ask that it be brought to the hospital and noted in her record. If the patient moves to another unit, make sure a copy of the directive goes with her.

It's important to remember that a patient can reverse either a consent to treatment or an advance directive, at any time; you should document any verbal comments that would change any previously expressed intent. Here are some other steps you can take to make the PSDA work better:

- Find out about your state's advance directive statute. For example, which life-sustaining measures are covered? Is there a time limit on the validity of a directive? Is it legal to follow a pregnant woman's documented wishes, even if doing so could endanger the fetus? In many states, it isn't.
- Speak to your risk manager, nursing administrator, or chaplain about your hospital's implementation of the PSDA. Are blank forms available—even though the law doesn't require this? Is a particular staff member or department responsible for helping patients fill them out? If not, suggest that these steps be taken, and that nurses become more involved. Also, find out if your state statute allows you to act as a witness for an advance directive.
- Look at the circumstances under which advance directives are discussed. The best place is in the attending physician's

office before a medical crisis arises. It's crucial that the subject of terminal care be raised while the patient is still competent, and that his preferences be recorded.

But that doesn't always happen. When the illness or injury is sudden, or a family in crisis is having trouble coming to terms with the decisions they must make, you need to be a good listener, as well as a source of information. You can also put the family in touch with chaplains, social workers, and members of the ethics committee, who can further assist with decision-making.

Help family members consider the idea that doing everything to keep a terminally ill patient alive isn't necessarily in his best interests. One way to do that is to ask, "If your loved one could speak to us now, what would he want?"

- Talk to your colleagues about end-of-life treatment choices. Encourage them to prepare their own advance directives. Work on becoming more comfortable discussing this issue with families and patients. Attend ethics conferences, if possible. And request that inservices be given on the subject if they're not provided; staff education is part of the PSDA mandate.

- Help your hospital get the word out to the community. As a nurse knowledgeable about end-of-life treatment issues, you can answer questions and help individuals make choices before they reach the hospital.

- Encourage patients to choose a proxy as well as preparing a living will. A person familiar with a patient's wishes about terminal care—and committed to respecting them—can be a better guide than a loosely worded living will.

For more information on advance directives, you can turn to these sources: American Health Decisions (319 E. 46th St., New York, NY 10017), Choice in Dying (250 W. 57th St., New York, NY 10019), and the Hastings Center, Institute of Society, Ethics, and the Life Sciences (255 Elm Rd., Briarcliff Manor, NY 10510).

New state laws extend the right to refuse treatment

Powerful as the PSDA seemed when it was passed, it has not been the ultimate answer. Two new kinds of laws address issues that either needed expansion or weren't addressed in the PSDA.

Surrogate decision-making statutes spell out, in order of priority, who is authorized to make decisions for an incompetent patient who hasn't made a living will or other directive. These laws help caregivers respect the wishes of family members or surrogates who act on behalf of a patient by reducing the fear of legal consequences.

The other type of new law addresses situations outside the hospital. Emergency personnel often begin CPR even when such life-saving efforts are futile, because that's what the law requires. Thus, the terminally ill patient who'd had DNR orders in the hospital is revived by the paramedics called by a panicked relative when he codes at home. To correct such situations, statutes recognizing "No CPR" documents give individuals the right to forego out-of-hospital resuscitation efforts. At present, though, only a few states have made these prehospital directives legal, and they apply only under certain restricted circumstances.

These new laws indicate a continuing trend toward greater respect for a patient's right to make vital health care decisions. But passing laws is one thing; changing attitudes is quite another. In this delicate and emotionally charged area, your active involvement on the side of the patient can often make the difference between honoring a person's last wishes and losing them in the shuffle.

Q&A:
Documentation
and Administration

Purging notes from the chart isn't an option

I charted a conversation I had with an exasperated mental health patient by quoting her complaints about the facility, including its sanitary conditions. My supervisor later asked me to remove my note from the chart and replace it with a vague statement such as "the patient expressed anger at the hospital setting." Was her request proper?

No. Notes in a patient's chart should never be removed or deleted, and especially not to make a person or institution look better. If the notes are erroneous or confusing, an addendum can be added to the chart to correct or clarify the record.

Moreover, there was nothing wrong with the way you charted in the first place. Complaints, abusive remarks, or other statements that you judge to be pertinent to a patient's condition and care—including that person's mental state or competence—should be documented. Any such statements should be charted verbatim to avoid subjective interpretations and vagueness.

If in doubt about what to include in a patient's record, consult your facility's risk management officer.

Second-hand verbal orders spell trouble

If I'm not around when a doctor telephones with orders, the instructions are relayed to me by whoever takes the call. What risks do I take when I act on orders transmitted by a third party, and how can I minimize them?

Communication errors are a frequent cause of patient injury—and a real possibility when verbal orders are passed from doctor to nurse via a third party. What's more, if the orders demand quick action, the time it takes to transmit the instructions could be costly to the patient's well-being.

Assuming the orders are not urgent, ask the person who spoke with the doctor to immediately document the order in the patient's record. By acting on the written orders, you'll at least avoid the possibility of misunderstanding a verbal communication that might not be relayed to you immediately and harming the patient as a result. If that's not an option, call the doctor back so you can speak with him directly.

Also, check your facility's policy and procedure manual. Most health care employers have strict policies on verbal orders, stipulating a time frame within which instructions must be charted by the nurse and signed off on by the physician.

What's an "incident"?

What constitutes an "incident" for the purposes of filling out an incident report?
Generally, it is any out-of-the ordinary event that involves potential or actual injury to a person, or potential or actual damage to property. It occurs within the hospital's network, including any satellite locations, or within the scope of the hospital's operations, such as during an ambulance transport provided by the facility.

Usually, a hospital provides a definition of "incident" or "occurrence" in its policy and procedure manual, so check that before filing a report. If in doubt, call the risk manager. When you are filling out the report, be sure to provide only factual information, not your opinions.

How to document home-safety checks

When doing a home-safety assessment, I use a check list supplied by my agency to document "safe" and "unsafe" conditions. Aren't these subjective terms? Shouldn't I avoid such judgments?
Absolutely, especially when it comes to describing household conditions. You're not an engineer, so you have no way of knowing whether, say, an electrical cord is "safe." What you can determine is whether the cord "appears intact" or is "not frayed," and these are the kind of objective terms you should use when documenting any household condition.

Talk to your supervisor about redesigning your assessment form so that it is more accurate and specific. That way, if there turns out to be a defect or hazard in the home that results in harm to the patient, your documentation can prove that it was not observable.

Documenting emergency transfers

My emergency department frequently transfers patients to a better-equipped hospital that's several miles away. When we are swamped, we don't always get our patients to sign a statement consenting to the transfer. How risky is this practice?

The Emergency Medical Treatment and Active Labor Act (EMTALA), commonly known as the anti-dumping law, applies to hospitals that receive federal funds. It requires health care facilities to stabilize all patients who present to the emergency department in unstable condition before transferring them to another facility, unless an immediate transfer is medically necessary.

Whenever an unstable patient is transferred to another facility, a physician at the first hospital must certify in writing that the benefits of care at the second facility outweigh the risks of delaying the patient's treatment.

The Emergency Medical Treatment and Active Labor Act also requires that you inform the patient or a member of his family of the benefits and risks of transfer, whenever that is possible. To prove that you've done that, ask the patient to sign a consent-to-transfer form or, if he doesn't want to be transferred, an informed refusal form.

If there is no signed statement and a lawsuit results, a court will look for other evidence that the patient was informed. You'll have a convincing case if you have documented in the chart that the risks and benefits of the transfer were explained to the patient, the names of anyone who witnessed the conversation, and the patient's response. Since you are required to notify the receiving facility to make arrangements for the transfer, document this contact as well.

Negligence charges don't belong in a chart

When a patient of mine fell getting out of bed, her physician charted that the incident was the result of "lax nursing supervision." What are the legal implications of such accusatory documentation?

Not good—for either you or the doctor. The medical record is one of the first places a plaintiff's attorney looks when investigating a charge of improper care. It is not the proper place for a physician or a nurse to comment on circumstances surrounding an accident—that should be done in an incident report. The charge could give a lawyer ammunition against you, the doctor, and the hospital.

Although the notation can't be deleted, don't compound the problem by addressing it in the chart. Instead, discuss the incident with the doctor, pointing out that it's improper to chart allegations about caregivers.

Tell your supervisor about the incident, too. She may want to inform an administrator or the hospital's risk manager.

How to chart hearsay

When I questioned a colleague about a patient's fall that she had detailed in his chart, she told me she had not actually seen the event but had been told about it by another nurse. Is it acceptable to chart something you didn't witness?

If an incident occurs that directly relates to the health and well-being of the patient, it is better to chart it yourself than to have it go undocumented. But first you should verify the information with a witness. If that individual is a professional caregiver, though, it is her legal duty to chart it.

If that's not possible—say, the witness has left the hospital—go ahead and chart the incident, but clearly present it as hearsay. For example, write "Gerri Michaels, RN, said the patient fell while getting out of bed."

If a patient won't give up her jewelry

A patient I'm caring for insists on keeping her diamond bracelet with her. How can I protect myself from liability if a patient's valuables are stolen? Most facilities have policies requiring that patients store valuables in the hospital safe or send them home. If a patient won't comply, document exactly what she insists on keeping and that she's keeping it with her despite your advice. Have her sign a form waiving any claim against the hospital if her belongings disappear. If your hospital doesn't have a such a form—or a valuables policy—ask your supervisor about developing one.

When you document valuables, use objective terms and avoid making judgments about authenticity. For instance, rather than labeling something a "diamond," describe it as a "clear stone."

Legal risks of poor penmanship

A physician at my hospital has illegible handwriting, so I usually rewrite his orders so the nurses I work with are able to read them. Is that proper?
No, and it's risky. For one thing, you may be misinterpreting the doctor's orders. If you jot down the wrong medication or dose, for example—either because you misread what's written or failed to copy it correctly—you could be harming the patient and setting yourself up for a negligence claim.

You could be charged with practicing medicine without a license, too. Unlike transcribing a verbal order, where you can ask the doctor for clarification, here you are interpreting illegible instructions on your own. Stop this practice immediately. Insist that the doctor either write legibly, print clearly, type, or dictate his orders instead.

Who's accountable for inadequate staffing?

I work in med/surg, but my DON wants me to cover our ED for four hours of my shift. This leaves three nurses caring for the med/surg patients, one of whom is on telemetry. None of these nurses has training in telemetry interpretation; I do. If something happens to the telemetry patient while I'm covering the ED, could I be held responsible?
The DON is responsible for staffing decisions, but only if she is apprised of patient needs by each nursing unit. Since it's her job to know her staff's professional skills, your obligation is to make her aware of the telemetry patient and his special needs. You can do that by noting it in your written shift report to the DON. As a staff nurse, you are then obligated to follow her directions, and cannot be held liable for poor decision-making on her part.

When a code jeopardizes proper staffing

As a charge nurse, I'm part of the code team at my hospital. The nursing supervisor is supposed to cover the staff on my unit when I'm participating in a code, but her services are usually needed during the resuscitation. Is it proper to leave the LPNs on my unit alone? And am I accountable for what happens on the unit in my absence?
Having neither a charge nurse, a supervisor, nor a staff RN on hand exposes patients to danger, especially if the unit has a high acuity level. LPNs don't have the same scope of practice that RNs have, and might not notice important changes in a patient's condition. If a patient sustains an injury during the time you and your supervisor are away, a claim of abandonment could be made.

The hospital, not you, is ultimately responsible for adequate staffing at all times to ensure quality patient care. Nonetheless, you are obligated to notify your employer about any potentially unsafe situation.

Talk to your department head about the lack of coverage during codes and the need for a policy to address this problem—such as a mechanism for pulling in a temporary supervisor. If you don't get a satisfactory response, put your concern in writing and take it up the chain of command.

If taking breaks hinders patient safety

Since our hospital became smoke-free, a co-worker asks me to cover her patients whenever she ducks outside for a cigarette. Could I be liable if one of her patients were injured during that time even though I've been stuck with a double load?

Yes. Whenever you cover a colleague's patients, regardless of the reason, you are still expected to meet the standard of care of a reasonably prudent nurse. However, your unit should provide safeguards for such instances—sufficient staff to cover for a nurse on break, for example, and protocols that require the staffer who is stepping outside to give report to the nurse covering for her. A nurse who walks off the unit without doing that is not being reasonably prudent—and could very well be held liable if a problem were to develop.

That would not let you off the hook, though: It is your responsibility to insist on being briefed before you take over another nurse's duties, even if it's only for a short time.

If your co-worker is taking an excessive number of breaks or stepping out without notice, talk to her about it. If her behavior continues, protect both yourself and her patients by bringing the matter to the attention of your supervisor.

Short-staffing: risky for staff and patients

I work in a rural hospital with a chronic nursing shortage, and at times I have as many as 11 patients. When two patients went into cardiac arrest recently, the DON criticized me for not having anticipated the emergency. Could I be liable for errors despite such a heavy load?

The fact that you're overloaded doesn't protect you from liability. But there are things you can do to bolster your defense in the event of a malpractice suit. First, file a written protest with the hospital administrator. Note your concerns about whether you can safely care for so many patients and ask for support staff. Be aware that your hospital has a duty to provide sufficient personnel and adhere to staffing ratios set by accrediting bodies or state agencies.

Keep a copy of the memo for your records. If you get no response, take your complaint up the chain of command. If you are assigned again to a unit where you feel the staffing is not adequate for the patients' acuity level, inform your supervisor about your concerns before you begin your shift.

If nothing changes, you may want to consider transferring to another setting in which short-staffing is not likely to be so acute. In the meantime, be sure you have ample malpractice insurance.

If you hear rumors about a colleague

I heard through a friend of a friend that a nurse at my hospital has a serious drinking problem. What's my duty in a situation like this?
If you were the nurse's supervisor, it would be incumbent on you to investigate the rumors by contacting those who have direct knowledge of the situation. But since you are not her supervisor, it's not appropriate for you to do or say anything— especially since heavy drinking at home doesn't necessarily affect job performance.

Well-intentioned second-hand reports can do as much damage to a person's reputation as intentional false accusations. For that reason, nonsupervisory personnel should report only facts of which they have first-hand, personal knowledge.

If a patient mistakes someone for a nurse

I recently overheard a patient mistakenly call a medical technician "Nurse" and then ask her a question. The technician answered—without correcting the patient's misimpression. Are there legal implications to that?
It depends. If the patient asked for directions to the bathroom, for example, there would have been no need to correct the mistake. However, if the patient asked about an issue that a nurse

needed to respond to, the technician should have identified her role or position, and referred the patient to a nurse.

If, instead, she answered the question without identifying herself, she could be charged with intentionally misrepresenting her credentials. That's not only illegal but also potentially harmful to the patient, who may act on incorrect information given by the "nurse."

Nurses across the country are concerned about unlicensed personnel misrepresenting themselves as RNs. But no health care worker—licensed or not—should be answering clinical questions that are outside the scope of her practice.

When the impaired nurse is your boss

I suspect that my supervisor has a drug problem, even though I do not have any hard evidence. I am concerned about the safety of patients— but also my job. What should I do?

Some states require you to report professional misconduct. If you live in one of them, you have little choice. The American Nurses Association's *Code of Ethics* also requires nurses to take steps to protect patients from coming to harm at the hands of an impaired colleague. So you are ethically bound to report an impaired co-worker, as well.

Because it is risky to accuse your supervisor of something, though, discreetly talk to your co-workers to see if they have been entertaining the same suspicions. It's generally safer to act in concert, and checking with others can help verify or negate your concerns.

If no one else thinks that your supervisor has a substance abuse problem, you should consider a course of watchful waiting: The signs of drug addiction are usually apparent to more than one person.

If your colleagues share your suspicions, however, or if you have a valid reason to believe that your supervisor could be endangering patients, set up a meeting with her boss right away.

Be certain that you stick with the facts and be careful not to make any statements that could be construed as being accusatory or defamatory.

Be careful if you are thinking of confronting your supervisor; if she is addicted, she may not be ready to deal with the problem herself.

Mental impairment and informed consent

In the endoscopy department where I work it's my job to have patients sign an informed consent form. We recently had a patient with senile dementia, whom I felt didn't fully understand the procedure he'd be having. Can someone with his condition give consent?

A mental condition like dementia or Alzheimer's doesn't automatically disqualify a patient from giving consent. The patient just has to be lucid at the time he does so.

It is ultimately the physician's responsibility to judge the patient's competence and adequately inform him about the procedure, its risks, and alternatives. However, if you have any doubts about the patient's understanding or competence—based on questions you've asked him—you must refrain from asking for his signature and inform the doctor.

Organ requests: what to tell families

A deceased patient's wife agreed to donate her husband's corneas when a nurse asked her to, but I don't think the woman had any idea that her husband's eyes would have to be removed. Is it permissible to leave out such information when obtaining consent for donations?

No. Nurses who approach families about organ donation have a legal, moral, and ethical duty to accurately represent if and how the deceased's body will be altered. If the nurse isn't sure exactly what will be harvested or what degree of disfigurement there will be, she should tell the family member so and then find out the information so a truly informed consent can be obtained.

Consent for postmortem teaching

Clinicians at my hospital routinely instruct staff by intubating recently deceased patients—without the consent of their next of kin. Is that legal? Interfering with a body before an autopsy may alter evidence in a legal case. There are local ordinances regarding the proper handling and disposal of a corpse. However, to our knowledge there is no law that requires family consent to perform instructional procedures.

From a legal perspective, intubation is different from organ harvesting, which requires the consent of the next of kin. A family could sue for emotional distress if they learned that intubation was performed on a dead relative without their okay, but the outcome of such a claim is uncertain.

Ideally, your hospital should have a policy regarding post mortem procedures, which also addresses ethical issues. If you feel that family consent should be required or have other ideas about what such a policy should include, discuss the matter with your supervisor or risk manager.

Rights and Responsibilities

If you're injured by a patient

You're cautioned constantly about the risk of being sued by a patient who's injured while under your care. But what if a patient injures you?

A nurse is responsible for the safety of her patient. But what recourse does a nurse have if he or she is injured by a patient? Since all nurses face aggressive or disoriented patients sometimes, it's a question every nurse ought to be able to answer. You may have options under both criminal and civil law.

If a patient threatens or intentionally hurts you, you have the right to press criminal charges, just as you would if a person threatened or assaulted you on the street. If you decide to press charges, notify the police as soon as possible after the situation has been defused and you've completed an incident report. After the police conduct an investigation, the district attorney's office will decide whether or not to prosecute the case.

If you need medical treatment or are unable to work as a result of your injuries—whether they were inflicted intentionally or not—you are entitled to workers' compensation. Depending on the circumstances of the case, you may also have grounds for filing a civil suit against the patient, seeking monetary compensation.

Hopefully, you won't have reason to explore either of these two options. But if you do, you should know what's entailed in each, the limitations of each, and the outcome of recent court cases.

An "innocent" touch leads to injury

The following case, decided in 1996 by the Wisconsin Supreme Court,[1] provides a glimpse into the thinking of the courts when it comes to personal injury claims filed by nurses.

Ronald Monicken, diagnosed with Alzheimer's disease, was institutionalized at St. Croix Health Care Center in Wisconsin. He was frequently disoriented and sometimes combative. He often wandered into the rooms of other patients and sometimes resisted when staff came to remove him.

On one such occasion, Sheri Gould, head nurse of the center's dementia unit, attempted to redirect Monicken to his own room by touching him on the elbow. He responded by knocking her to the ground, injuring her.

Gould sued Monicken and his insurer, American Family Mutual Insurance Company, for damages. At trial, the jury was instructed to disregard Monicken's mental condition in deciding whether he was guilty of negligence in injuring Gould. The jury found that Monicken had indeed been negligent.

American Family appealed, arguing that Monicken could not be held liable because his mental condition made him incapable of controlling his conduct.

When the case reached the Wisconsin high court, it agreed. The court ruled that holding Monicken negligent would place too great a burden on him because his disorientation and potential for violence was the very reason he was institutionalized and needed professional care.

In addition, the court said, "When a mentally disabled person injures an employed caretaker, the injured party can reasonably foresee the danger and is not 'innocent' of the risk involved." In this case, Gould had express knowledge of the danger inherent in dealing with Alzheimer's patients in general and Monicken in particular.

Consequently, the court held that a person institutionalized with a mental disability who does not have the capacity to control or appreciate his behavior cannot be held liable for injuries caused to caretakers who are employed for monetary compensation.

When can the patient be held accountable?

While state laws on civil liability vary, the Wisconsin case illustrates how the ability to sue successfully may depend on a couple of key factors: whether the risk of harm from the patient was foreseeable and whether the patient was mentally competent at the time.

In certain situations, like caring for mentally impaired patients, courts may consider the risk of being struck by a patient an expected part of a nurse's job, much like the risk of being burned is part of a firefighter's. Because providing care during risky patient interactions may be the very reason a nurse is needed—and part of what she gets paid for—courts may view it as unfair to hold the patient liable if he injures that nurse.

There's another, but similar, line of legal thinking: Employees who knowingly expose themselves to such risk presumably have the skills, knowledge, and resources to avoid injury. If they're unable to do so and subsequently sue, the defense may ask the jury to consider whether the incident was at least partly the result of the employee's own actions.

In the Wisconsin case, for example, you could argue the nurse should have known that suddenly touching an aggressive and disoriented patient on the elbow could trigger his combative reflexes.

As for the relevance of the patient's mental state, in most jurisdictions common law has long held that individuals are responsible for their actions regardless of their mental capacity. But within the last two decades, some courts have started to carve out exceptions to that rule.

They've taken into account, for example, whether the defendant was able to control and understand the consequences of his behavior, and whether the behavior was of his own making—particularly if that person was under professional care. If, say, a patient strikes a nurse after being given a medication that caused him to become delirious, no court is likely to hold that patient accountable.

It should be noted that civil suits generally aren't filed unless the plaintiff sustained a serious or permanent injury that resulted in pain or suffering. The benefit of suing in such cases is that it can result in far more monetary compensation than workers' comp affords. (Workers' comp benefits are discussed below.) But, there is a downside.

For one thing, your own behavior will be scrutinized to see if you contributed to or even provoked the incident. Secondly, many patients do not have the assets to pay out a judgment, and may not have an insurance policy that provides personal liability coverage. So you'll wind up with nothing even if a jury finds in your favor.

In many states, coverage for an injury caused by a person's acts is provided under that person's homeowners' or rental policy, even if those acts occur beyond the premises. However, such policies usually disclaim coverage for intentional harm, instead covering only acts of negligence—in which the insured person did not act in a reasonable and prudent manner.

If you ever need to consider suing, it's best to discuss the merits of your case with an attorney who specializes in personal injury claims.

Workers' comp: There for the asking

As a rule, workers' compensation covers injuries caused by accidents arising out of and in the course of employment. That would include any injury caused by a patient, provided that you were acting within the scope of your employment at the time.

Because workers' compensation is a type of "no fault" insurance, it doesn't matter if your own negligence or that of your employer caused or contributed to your injury. Your employer can't hold you accountable and you can't sue your employer. You do, however, retain the right to sue a third party, like a patient.

As long as you are in an employer-employee relationship, you are probably covered by workers' comp. Nurses who are independent contractors technically work for themselves, and therefore are not covered. Private duty and per diem nurses who get their own assignments fall into this category. Also, in a few states, employers with only a small number of employees—say, fewer than four—are not required to provide coverage.

The amount and duration of benefits vary by state, and there's a separate compensation plan that applies to federal employees. The basic items covered, though, are the same. All medical and hospital bills arising from the job-related injury are covered, provided they are for treatments approved by your employer's workers' comp carrier.

If you're temporarily disabled, most states compensate for lost wages with weekly payments of two-thirds your usual wage. Most states, however, set a dollar limit that may be much lower than that level.

For a permanent total or partial impairment, you are also entitled to a flat award based on the type of disability. If you will never be able to return to work, the settlement is based on your loss of earning power and physical or mental limitations. Unlike awards made in a civil case, there are no awards for pain and suffering with workers' comp.

To ensure you get what coverage you are entitled to, submit a detailed written report of the incident to your supervisor as soon as possible after it occurs. Follow your employer's accident reporting procedures. Do this even if you're not sure that you'll require medical treatment—seemingly minor injuries can turn into major ones.

Be aware that if you receive money through workers' comp and later win money in a civil suit, you will have to reimburse your employer's workers' comp carrier for the benefits that the carrier paid you.

Certainly, an element of risk comes with the nursing territory. If that risk should ever become a reality, you owe it to yourself to see that you're compensated to the maximum that the law allows.

REFERENCES

1. Gould and St. Croix County v. American Family Mutual Insurance Company, 198 Wis. 2d 450, 1996.

When assignments don't match skills

Accepting an assignment you don't feel qualified for can lead to a liability suit; refusing it could end in dismissal. Here's how to walk the middle ground.

At the surgeon's request, an OR nurse applies cricoid pressure to a patient, a procedure she had been taught to do only once, a year before. While reaching down to get a piece of equipment, she momentarily releases the pressure—not knowing it's dangerous to do so. The patient immediately vomits and aspirates gastric contents. Postop, the patient's condition deteriorates, and she dies a few weeks later.[1]

When a nurse or other health care worker is asked to perform a task she's not properly trained to do, the consequences can be deadly to the patient, costly to the hospital—the OR nurse's employer paid a half-million-dollar settlement—and devastating to the individual's career.

For health professionals who delegate work, including nurse supervisors, charge nurses, and staff RNs who oversee unlicensed assistive personnel (UAPs), the price of making an inappropriate assignment can be equally high.

But it's not just performing or assigning complex procedures that nurses have to worry about. Floating to unfamiliar units, an increasingly common practice in light of stepped-up staff reductions, raises concerns about patient safety and professional liability, too.

With good reason. Simply saying No to an assignment that makes you uncomfortable is rarely an option. Unless you have a contract or written agreement that spells out your duties and the unit you'll work on, your employer can generally dictate what you do and where you do it. But there are times when you're entitled, even obligated, to refuse to go along.

Basing your refusal on solid grounds

When you are given an assignment you believe you're unsuited for, find out precisely what your duties will be and how much supervision you will receive. You will need to weigh your level of skill and training against the riskiness of the procedure or the acuity of the patients you would be caring for.

The interests of the patients should be the determinant in deciding whether to accept the assignment. For example, floating to a unit in a specialty you know nothing about isn't optimal, but if the unit is short-staffed and no other nurse is available it might be the safest option for the patients.

Remember, the legal system does not expect your nursing care to be perfect—just consistent with that provided by a reasonably prudent nurse with similar training and expertise under similar circumstances. However, you do have to put the person giving you the assignment on notice of potential problems by voicing any reservations you have. (We'll explain the best way to do that in the next section.)

There are two documents that provide you with unquestionable grounds for refusing an assignment. The first is your employee manual, which should spell out hospital policy and procedure. A student nurse, for example, may be prohibited from performing certain tasks without direct supervision. If you're asked to do something contrary to policy or procedure, refuse.

The second shield is your state's nurse practice act; refuse to perform any task not permitted by it. In some states, for example, enterostomal nurses are allowed to do wound debridement;

in others they are not. If you're not sure whether a particular task or procedure is beyond your scope of practice, contact the state board of nursing. If you have time, do so before beginning the assignment; if you don't, let your supervisor know about your doubts and the fact that you'll be checking.

Express reservations, then explore alternatives

Often, though, your reason for not wanting an assignment will be subjective, based on your belief that you lack sufficient training or experience, for instance. A lot of nurses, especially new grads, talk themselves out of these concerns rather than question their superior's judgment. That's a mistake.

If you are asked to perform a technical function you feel is beyond your training or experience, discuss your reservations with either the person making the request or your supervisor. In an emergency situation, there may not be time for this. But when you can, state your case in factual terms rather than emotional ones. Be as specific as possible.

For example, instead of saying, "I'm not comfortable taking care of ventilator patients," say "I've cared for ventilator patients only a few times but never without close supervision," or "The last time I did this was several years ago, and with different equipment."

Express a willingness to fill patient care needs in a capacity you do feel comfortable with: Do ancillary duties rather than act as charge nurse, for example.

Request that the assignment be delayed until you receive appropriate inservicing or cross-training. Any time you're offered such training, you'd be wise to accept the offer. The case of an ICU nurse who refused to float to an orthopedics unit because he didn't feel qualified to act as the charge nurse there makes that message clear: The hospital offered to orient him, but he declined and was later terminated. In ruling for the hospital in this wrongful discharge suit, the New Mexico Supreme Court noted that the nurse's unwillingness to take orientation or even try working in orthopedics undermined his case.[2]

If your supervisor won't change your assignment despite your objections, you have two choices: Refuse it and risk disciplinary action, or accept the assignment and prepare yourself as much as you can.

If you choose the latter, learn all you can about your new assignment. For instance, find out what the chain of command is, which doctors to contact if necessary, and, of course, what you will be responsible for on a unit you've never worked on before. Speak with the nurse supervisor and charge nurse beforehand about getting whatever assistance you feel you need.

Whenever you refuse an assignment or accept it under duress, document your reasons or objections. Fill out an "assignment under protest" form, available from some state nurses associations. Or write a memo of your own. Stick to the facts, listing the specific tasks you were asked to do and the reasons you are not qualified. Include the name of the individual to whom you expressed your objections.

Give copies of the memo to your immediate supervisor, the person who gave you the assignment, and an appropriate administrator. Keep a copy for yourself. If you're given a similar assignment a second time—but no additional training or preparation—take your concerns up the chain of command.

Minimize risks when you make the assignment

Caution is the watchword, too, on the other side of the fence. Anyone who delegates could be found negligent for making an inappropriate or unsafe assignment if the patient is harmed as a result.

As long as you act with reasonable prudence—assigning a function within the staffer's scope of training and providing a level of supervision commensurate with the staffer's skill and patient's condition—you probably won't be held liable if the individual is negligent. It is quite a different story if you don't exercise reasonable foresight and oversight, as the following case highlights:

An inexperienced nurse working the night shift was assigned to an acutely ill patient. When the patient developed signs of respiratory distress, the nurse telephoned the attending specialist rather than the hospital's emergency physician. She then left the patient unattended for several minutes while she waited for the specialist to call. The patient went into respiratory arrest and died shortly thereafter.[3]

The hospital had to pay about $2.5 million in damages. The plaintiff's lawyers had a lot to work with: The records revealed that not only was a nurse just out of school assigned to a seriously ill patient, but the two other nurses on duty had provided woefully inadequate oversight, neither monitoring her closely nor making sure she knew how to proceed in an emergency.

To avoid such disasters, make sure that you are familiar with the skills and abilities of any staffer you supervise or to whom you assign work. Arrange for an appropriate degree of monitoring and, if necessary, collaboration with other nurses. Delay potentially problematic tasks to other shifts if possible. Review staffing patterns in advance to fill gaps where needed.

If inadequate staffing or other conditions force you to make assignments you believe to be unsafe or prevent you from properly overseeing work, put somebody on notice: Contact your supervisor or an administrator before making the assignment. Then document your concerns in a memo. Remember, state agencies and the Joint Commission require hospitals—not employees—to ensure safe staffing levels.

Avoid future problems by developing criteria for assigning work based on evaluations of staffers' clinical skills. Develop a plan for cross-training nurses to sister units. Request cross-training for yourself, so it's less likely you'll have to challenge an assignment you could have been prepared to accept.

REFERENCES

1. Rubsamen, D. S. (Ed.). (1994). A fatal case of aspiration pneumonitis. Professional Liability Newsletter, 24(10).
2. David W. Francis v. Memorial General Hospital, 726 P. 2d 852 (1986). Supreme Court of New Mexico.
3. Rubsamen, D. S. (Ed.). (1993). The inexperienced nurse and a $2.6 million settlement. Professional Liability Newsletter, 23(10).

You don't have to care for every patient

You have the right to refuse an assignment that conflicts with your personal values. But there's a right way to say No.

A
bortion. Withdrawal of nutrition and hydration. Sterilization. These and other procedures may raise profound ethical issues for the nurses who have to participate in them.

The ANA's *Code for Nurses* upholds the right of nurses to refuse any assignment they ethically oppose.[1] And in 1995, for the first time, the Joint Commission on Accreditation of Healthcare Organizations (JCAHO) acknowledged that right, too. It added a standard to both its hospital and home care accreditation manuals that requires employers to establish policies and mechanisms to address staff requests not to participate in aspects of care that conflict with cultural values or religious beliefs.

The JCAHO expanded upon that standard in its 1996 hospital accreditation manual, and did the same in its 1997 home care manual. The new hospital standard requires each facility to:[2]

■ Specify those aspects of patient care that might conflict with staff members' values or beliefs.

■ Have a written policy on how requests to be excused from care are handled and make that policy available to all staff.

■ Develop a process for deciding whether staff requests not to participate in care are legitimate and should be granted. In other words, nurses will not be automatically excused from an assignment just because they say it conflicts with their cultural values, ethics, or religious beliefs.

■ Ensure the safe delivery of care in instances when a staff member's request to be excused is granted.

The JCAHO standard bolsters the rights of nurses whose beliefs may clash with certain aspects of care and supplements the legal protections that already exist for them. All nurses should know what those protections are, as well as the safe, proper way to decline assignments they personally oppose.

Religious protection, conscience clauses

The courts have generally upheld an employee's right to refuse to participate in a job function that conflicts with his or her religious beliefs. Discrimination in employment on the basis of religion is illegal under Title VII of the 1964 Civil Rights Act, and an employer must reasonably accommodate an employee's religious practices unless doing so would cause the employer undue hardship.

In one well-known case, Margaret Kenney, an OR nurse, was demoted after she objected on religious grounds to assisting in abortions. The court, finding that the majority of nursing duties at the employer's ambulatory center didn't involve gynecological procedures, stated that the center had a legal duty to accommodate Ms. Kenney's religious beliefs and ordered that she be reinstated to her former position.[3]

While Title VII offers the most sweeping protection for nurses who have religious objections to participating in certain care, "conscience clauses" often provide more explicit protection. Most states have such statutes[4] that protect health care personnel from reprisals if they refuse to participate in certain defined procedures. Most conscience clauses allow a refusal based on moral or ethical beliefs, not just religious ones.

For example, when nurse anesthetist Marjorie Swanson was fired after she refused to participate in a tubal ligation, she asserted her rights under the Montana conscience clause. The courts, stating that the clause prohibited firing any person for refusing to participate in sterilization on moral or religious grounds, ordered a trial to determine if Swanson's refusal was the reason for her discharge.[5]

Conscience clauses by no means offer blanket protection, though. Most protect only those employees who refuse to participate in abortions or sterilizations. A few state statutes do bestow broader protection. Maryland's, for instance, allows employees to refuse to participate in artificial insemination.

There is also a federal conscience clause, which applies to facilities that receive certain types of government funding—including grants under the Public Health Service Act and Community Mental Health Centers Act. Like those in most states, the federal clause prohibits only discrimination against staff who refuse to assist in sterilizations or abortions because of religious beliefs or moral convictions.[6]

Objections that uphold the public good

If you belong to a union and your employment contract specifies your job duties, your employer may not be able to require you to perform different duties—ones that you may be ethically opposed to. However, if you are not working under an employment contract, meaning that you are an at-will employee, the public policy exception to at-will employment may offer you some protection.

Under this doctrine, employers can't take actions against employees that would undermine a clearly defined public policy. For example, a nurse who's been fired for refusing to commit an illegal act or to violate the nurse practice act—such as by performing certain medical procedures at her employer's behest—may be able to win reinstatement.

Be aware, however, that not all states recognize the public policy exception. And, since the public policy doctrine looks toward protecting the public good, it is often construed narrowly. So, what may be objectionable to you personally, may not be objectionable in the eyes of the state legislature or court.

In one case, for instance, a nurse was fired for refusing to continue to dialyze a terminally ill double amputee who had suffered cardiac arrest and hemorrhage during the procedure. The nurse contended that she had acted in the public interest, arguing that language in the ANA ethics code —permitting nurses not to participate in care they personally oppose— constituted an expression of public policy. But both a trial court and appellate court disagreed.[7]

Avoid problems before they surface

You'll have a much better chance of avoiding disputes over matters of conscience if you make your position against performing certain types of procedures or care known in advance. Speak with your supervisor about your objections and request that you not be given those assignments that conflict with your deeply held beliefs.

If you're currently caring for a patient and a change in his condition suddenly warrants an aspect of care that you object to, it's important that you alert your supervisor or the appropriate person as soon as possible so that the patient can be reassigned or other alternate arrangements made. In the Swanson case— the nurse who refused to assist in a sterilization—part of the reason the court ruled that a trial should be held was because Swanson had notified her hospital of her refusal only hours before the procedure, an action the court questioned.

Be aware that once you begin treating a patient, you're legally responsible for him until he has been placed in the care of someone else. If you refuse to continue to care for him, you could be endangering the patient and facing an abandonment charge. What's more, in an emergency, you must provide treatment, regardless of any personal objections you may have.

In nonemergency situations, make sure you strictly follow your employer's policy and procedures for refusing assignments. Familiarize yourself with them now. Since the JCAHO standard on handling staff requests not to participate in care is relatively new, some hospitals and home care agencies may still be in the process of developing a policy; others may still be unaware of their obligations under the JCAHO standards, in which case you may want to enlighten them!

Whether your employer has a policy in place or not, if you decide not to be involved in an aspect of care, make crystal clear the grounds for your refusal. Conscience clauses, like many existing employer policies, require that the employee's objection be based on moral, ethical, or religious beliefs. So frame your refusal in those terms, and be explicit. You can't just say "I don't want to be involved in this."

If there is a dispute about the appropriateness of your refusal, you can request that the matter be brought to the hospital attorney, risk manager, or ethics committee. With the JCAHO standard providing new impetus, finding a solution that's agreeable to the nurse, the patient, and the employer should be that much easier.

REFERENCES

1. American Nurses Association. (1985). Code for nurses with interpretive statements. Kansas City, MO: Author.
2. Joint Commission. (1996). 1996 Accreditation manual for hospitals: Vol. 1, Standards. Oakbrook Terrace, IL: Joint Commission on Accreditation of Healthcare Organizations.
3. Kenney v. Ambulatory Center of Miami, Fla. App., 400 So. 2d 1262, 1981.
4. Vandecaveye, L. (1988, November). Employee rights in matters of conscience. Paper presented at the American Bar Association meeting, New Orleans.
5. Swanson v. St. John's Luehrs Hospital, 597 P.2d. 702, 1979.
6. Federal Conscience Clause, 42 U.S. Code, 3009.7.
7. Warthen v. Toms River Comm. Mem. Hosp. 488 A.2d 299, N.J. 1985.

If you question a doctor's orders

Nurses used to be fired for disagreeing with a doctor. Now the law is finally taking your side.

The young woman just admitted to your unit is vomiting and delirious with fever. When you assess her, you find her blood pressure dangerously low and her skin covered with a sunburn-like reddish rash. You suspect toxic shock syndrome—a massive bacterial infection that can cause death if it isn't treated right away.

You immediately report your findings to the doctor, certain she will order IV antibiotics at once. But she doesn't. When you bring the matter to your supervisor's attention, she tells you to stay out of it. By the time you are able to track down the hospital's chief of staff, who does intercede on the patient's behalf, it's too late. Your patient has died—from toxic shock syndrome.

Extremely upset by how this case was handled, you complain to several other nurses. Before you know it, you're hauled in by the hospital administrator, who fires you on the spot for making negative statements about hospital policies.

Your job is clear: Speak up for your patient

In years past, fears of scenarios like this were often enough to keep nurses subservient. With your greater professional stature and independence, however, you are now not only expected to stand up for standards of patient care, you're *required* to. And courts are backing you up.

In fact, the case posed above is based on an actual one in Missouri. A court of appeals—returning the case to a lower court for trial—ruled that the state's Nurse Practice Act makes it an "absolute duty" for nurses to speak up on behalf of their patients. Nurses who fulfill this obligation by challenging doctors' orders cannot be dismissed on these grounds, the court held. That's because "a clear mandate of public policy" makes this situation an exception to laws that otherwise allow employers to fire employees at will—whether or not there's reason.[1]

This precedent-setting case may go a long way toward resolving a dilemma many nurses still face—how to speak up for what you believe without putting your job or your career on the line.

One thing to remember is that the ANA code clearly states that it is a nurse's duty to advocate what is best for her patients. A nurse should act "to safeguard the client and the public when health care and safety are affected by the incompetent, unethical, or illegal practices of any person," the code says.[2]

State laws uphold your code of conduct

State nurse practice acts generally follow the ANA code. At least nine states—Delaware, Florida, New York, Minnesota, Rhode Island, Massachusetts, Nevada, Texas, and Oregon—also have laws requiring nurses to blow the whistle on incompetent medical acts. And their courts have upheld such laws, finding that nurses must inform their superiors if they feel a patient is not receiving proper care and they are unable to work it out with the attending doctor.[3]

What had not been sorted out prior to the Missouri case was whether a nurse who obeys such a law and openly challenges the authority of a doctor, supervisor, or her hospital could still lose her job.

In the Missouri case, which was resolved in 1993, the court said the answer was No, a nurse could not be dismissed for upholding her professional standards. If the decision serves as precedent in other states, it will add to the job protection nurses have gained over the years. In more than half the states, for instance, it is now unlawful for an employer to fire an employee who refuses to commit an illegal act—for example, falsifying or destroying patient records.[4]

If you are still worried about what may happen if you speak out, check with an employment attorney or your state nurses association to find out what actions are legally protected. No matter what the law, however, you can protect yourself and your patients by reporting any medical actions that you believe to be harmful.

But always go through the proper chain of command; most hospitals have a risk manager or quality assurance staff whose job it is to look into this kind of allegation. Talk to them first, and follow up, if necessary, in writing.

Think carefully, too, before you go public with a complaint. Bear in mind that it's legal for an employer to dismiss a nurse whose behavior is found by the courts to be "needlessly disruptive"—publicly challenging an administrative policy is an example.[5] Hospitals have a right to protect themselves against employees making frivolous or false accusations, so make sure you have good—and, if possible, documented—grounds for your complaint. To make sure you've got the facts right, check with other people who witnessed what you think was improper conduct to see if they agree with you.

If you work for a private hospital, your employer will have more leeway in its employment policies than public health care facilities do. But the Missouri case holds promise for all nurses, safeguarding your freedom to speak your mind on diagnosis- and treatment-related matters—without fear of retaliation.

REFERENCES

1. Kirk v. Mercy Hosp. Tri-County, 851 S.W.2d 617 - MO (1993).

2. American Nurses' Association (1976). American Nurses' Association code for nurses. Washington: American Nurses' Association.

3. Cushing, M. (1988). Nursing jurisprudence. East Norwalk, CT: Appleton & Lange.

4. Calloway, S. D., & Kota, J. M. (1989). Legal issues in supervising nurses (2nd ed.) Eau Claire, WI: Professional Education Systems.

5. Staff. (1990). Regan Report on Nursing Law, 30(9), 1.

The nurse's role in police investigations

Two cases highlight the legal risks for nurses when law enforcement officers bring criminal suspects to the hospital for blood tests.

There's nothing odd about a police officer escorting a suspect into the emergency department. Often, it's to have physical evidence collected—blood samples, for instance, in cases of suspected drunk driving or sexual assault.

Obtaining a physical specimen sounds straightforward enough. But two recent cases uncover some hidden, and unusual, legal issues when a suspect is brought to a hospital. In the first case, a nurse found herself caught between a rock and a hard place—faced with either having to disobey a court order or violate her professional and ethical standards. In the second, the question of whether a suspect is a "patient" became pivotal to deciding whether emergency department personnel had committed negligence.

A determined officer, an unwilling prisoner

One night in 1995 a New Jersey police sergeant brought a rape suspect to South Jersey Hospital–Millville and directed nurses in the ED to obtain blood specimens for a rape-kit analysis. When the suspect refused to allow his blood to be drawn and began to physically resist, the nurses contacted Marianne Robinson, RN, the house supervisor that night.

Robinson, after conferring with the administrator on call, John Lipson, MD, and hospital attorney Frank Ciesla, told the sergeant that the hospital staff would not draw blood from the suspect against his will. The sergeant left but was back a short while later—this time with a court order instructing unnamed hospital personnel to obtain the specimen, even if force was necessary.

Robinson again contacted Lipson, who spoke with Ciesla and the sergeant. According to Ciesla, the court order the police officer presented was unenforceable; it was not directed to any specific hospital and did not name the individuals who should draw the blood. In Ciesla's opinion, the hospital was not legally obligated to comply, and neither Robinson nor Lipson did.

Faced with South Jersey's continued refusal, the sergeant took the suspect to another medical center—which had an agreement with police to obtain specimens from suspects—and the sample was taken there.

Within days, warrants were issued charging Robinson and Lipson with obstructing the conduct of a law enforcement investigation and contempt of court. The two were told to report to police headquarters for fingerprinting and mug shots, an order that was dropped when Ciesla protested.

If convicted, Robinson and Lipson faced up to a year in jail.

Two sides to every story

The prosecutors who filed the charges maintained that health professionals in New Jersey are required under state law to assist police in obtaining bodily substances from suspects. The law gives nurses, physicians, medical technicians, and hospitals immunity from civil and criminal liability provided the specimen is taken in a "medically accepted manner."[1] Prosecutors also maintained that hospital personnel had no right to disobey a court order.

The hospital, meanwhile, filed suit against the county prosecutor and the Millville police department, seeking to prevent them from ordering the hospital to draw blood from unwilling suspects in the future. The New Jersey Hospital Association (NJHA) and the Medical Society of New Jersey filed court briefs in support of the hospital's position.

The medical society argued that while state law encourages cooperation between health care professionals and police, it does not mandate it. Furthermore, the qualified immunity statute doesn't provide adequate protection for health care personnel.

The NJHA contended, among other things, that a hospital and its employees have no obligation—indeed no right—to take physical specimens from a nonconsenting suspect. Subjecting an individual to invasive treatment against his will goes against established law, which gives competent adults the right to accept or reject health care interventions.

A medical professional who uses force to take a specimen, the NJHA argued, is deviating from his legal and ethical obligation to do no harm. The NJHA also pointed out that the police had other avenues for obtaining the blood sample, such as taking the suspect to a state or county prison medical facility.

A New Jersey superior court judge ruled in favor of the hospital, finding that the state law does not require hospitals to obtain bodily samples from suspects against their will.

Despite the ruling, the charges against the nurse and physician remained pending for months before prosecutors decided to drop them.

Suspect or patient? The line gets blurry

While Robinson and Lipson faced criminal prosecution because they refused to comply with an order to draw blood, the hospital in this next case faced a civil suit after one of its health care workers did comply with a police request to obtain a blood sample.

John Gooch was stopped by a state trooper after he was seen driving erratically on a West Virginia highway. His speech was slurred, he had trouble with his balance and coordination, and he failed a field sobriety test. Gooch told the state trooper that he had not been drinking but was taking several medications.[2]

Gooch had, in fact, seen a doctor the previous day about a respiratory condition. The doctor had given him an injection of penicillin and vitamin B_{12} and a prescription for penicillin pills.

The trooper didn't find any medication in Gooch's car. He did find an open bottle of whiskey, though, and arrested Gooch for driving under the influence.

Gooch agreed to have a blood test to determine the presence of drugs or alcohol and was taken to Raleigh General Hospital where a medical technologist drew the sample. He was then taken to county jail and released the following day.

Two days later Gooch died of strep pneumonia. The blood test came back negative for drugs or alcohol.

Gooch's family sued the hospital, alleging that it was liable for his death because the staff had failed to recognize that Gooch was not drunk but sick. The hospital, in seeking summary judgment, argued that it could not possibly be liable, since no hospital-patient relationship had ever been established.

The court agreed with the hospital, ruling that this type of relationship only exists if a person receives, or should have received, health care services. Simply bringing an arrested person to a hospital for a blood test, the court held, is not enough to create a hospital-patient relationship.

The court noted the fact that emergency department personnel had no reason to believe that Gooch was ill and in need of medical attention; neither Gooch nor the trooper had mentioned this possibility. If Gooch had requested medical services or if there was reason to believe he needed any, hospital personnel would have been required to perform medical screening and treatment as required under the Emergency Medical Treatment and Active Labor Act (EMTALA).[2]

Protecting yourself by playing it safe

As these two cases illustrate, you may face legal repercussions whether you agree to obtain a specimen from a suspect or refuse to do so. But there are ways to guard against the possibility of legal action.

First, because state laws vary, be familiar with your state's statute regarding the collection of physical evidence at the request of law enforcement. Most states provide immunity to health care facilities and personnel who draw blood at the direction of a police officer, as long as they do so properly. Immunity does not extend to cases of gross negligence or wanton or willful injury.[3]

Although most states do not require that police requests for blood tests be made in writing, attorneys recommend that you ask the officer to complete and sign a hospital form. Also ask the person who is having blood drawn to sign a consent form. The form should state explicitly the reason the blood is being drawn—for example, to determine alcohol content.[3]

If the person refuses to give consent but the police officer orders you to draw blood anyway, consult your hospital attorney or supervisor about how to proceed. "Most states require a court order to draw blood over a patient's refusal," says Donnaline Richman, RN, JD, a health law attorney with the firm Fager & Amsler in Syracuse, N.Y. Even then, the hospital may dispute the validity of the order, as the hospital in Millville, N.J. did.

When a police officer brings a suspect to the ED, attorneys advise that you ask the person if he or she requires any health care services, and document that you have done so. If the answer is No, and based on your observations or what you've been told you have no reason to believe that medical aid is needed, then it's clear that no hospital-patient relationship has been established.[3]

Richman recommends, however, that you go one step further. "Perform triage to determine if a screening exam is necessary. Diabetes or another medical problem may be the cause of erratic driving. Ask any person brought in for a driving-while-intoxicated test if, what, and how much he drank and if he's on any meds." Of course, the patient is entitled to refuse screening tests or medical services, but again, document any such refusal.

Every hospital should have a policy in place that spells out procedures to be taken when police bring suspects to the ED. If yours doesn't, speak with your risk manager or supervisor about developing one. Richman also suggests that hospital personnel meet with the local police to get potential problems resolved in advance and to educate them about the hospital's policy.

A clash of interests is always a possibility when police, suspects, and health care professionals must interact. Awareness and preparation are perhaps the best tools for harmonizing those interests when possible, and minimizing the likelihood of liability when it's not.

REFERENCES

1. N.J. Stat. 2A:62A-10 (1994).
2. Gooch v. West Virginia Department of Public Safety, 1995 W. Va. LEXIS 213.
3. Horty, Springer & Mattern, P.C. (December 1995/January 1996). Hospital duty to those arrested for DUI. Patient Care Law, p. 3.

If you're sexually harassed

Sexual harassment demands decisive action. It helps knowing that the force of the law will be behind you.

Several years ago, the Clarence Thomas hearings brought sexual harassment smack into people's living rooms. Although sexual harassment has yet to be eliminated from the workplace, an increasing number of victims are fighting back.

Nearly 16,000 sexual harassment claims were filed with the Equal Employment Opportunity Commission (EEOC) in 1995—two-and-a-half times the number filed in 1990.[1] That same year, employers paid out about $24 million in EEOC administrative settlements to victims of sexual harassment.[1]

Although males as well as females are sexually harassed, 90% of the claims filed with the EEOC are brought by women. That's not surprising, according to Elaine Herskowitz, JD, a senior attorney with the EEOC's Office of Legal Counsel: "Sexual harassment is typically perpetrated by people who have power over their victims. And men are more often in a position of power."

That's especially so in health care—and one reason nurses may be particularly vulnerable to sexual harassment. Another is that health care employees often develop close working relationships because of the intense nature of their work.[2] Thus, usual social constraints between professionals may become relaxed, making sexual innuendo and inappropriate behavior more likely. What's more, the human body and sexuality are legitimate, even necessary, topics of conversation among health care professionals.[2]

Surveys of nurses hint at the scope of the problem. In one study 46% of 188 critical care nurses reported being sexually harassed.[3] In another, 72% of 79 hospital-based RNs said they had been harassed.[4]

What, exactly, is sexual harassment?

For one thing, sexual harassment is a violation of Title VII of the Civil Rights Act, which bans sexual discrimination in workplaces with at least 15 employees. Fair employment statutes—which exist in most states and may apply to settings with fewer than 15 employees—usually prohibit sexual harassment, too.

The EEOC, which enforces Title VII, defines sexual harassment as unwanted sexual advances, requests for sexual favors, and other verbal or physical conduct of a sexual nature. Such conduct is either put on a quid-pro-quo basis or creates a hostile work environment.

Quid-pro-quo harassment exists when a superior, either implicitly or explicitly, makes submission to sexual demands a condition of employment or the basis for employment decisions.

A hostile environment exists when someone's unwelcome sexual conduct is pervasive or severe enough to intimidate or offend an employee, or to interfere with her ability to do her job. Whether the harasser actually intended to create a hostile environment isn't relevant. What matters is that the victim perceived it as such, and that a reasonable person would too.

Until a few years ago, employees who claimed that a hostile work environment had been created had to prove that the conduct of the harasser caused them severe psychological injury. In 1993, however, the United States Supreme Court unanimously held that the conduct need not seriously affect an employee's psychological well-being. "Title VII comes into play before the harassing conduct leads to a nervous breakdown," wrote Justice Sandra Day O'Connor in the high court's opinion.[5]

And what constitutes a hostile environment? That determination is based on any number of factors, including frequency of the conduct, its severity, and whether it is physically threatening. No single factor is required.

Lewd jokes, sexual comments, displays of suggestive material, or repeated requests for dates may all constitute a hostile environment, according to attorney Barbara Sapin, JD, general counsel at the ANA. In some cases, a single, traumatic event, such as a physical assault, may be enough to establish a hostile environment.

What should you do if you're harassed?

Experts agree that the best course of action is to confront the harasser and state clearly and unequivocally that the attention is unwanted. If you are in a union, ask your labor representative to accompany you, suggests Sapin. That person may be able to put a stop to the conduct simply by telling the harasser that the behavior is illegal.

Depending on the severity of the harassment and the person who's doing it, direct confrontation may be too difficult for you. If that's the case, at least "make sure you are not sending mixed signals," advises the EEOC's Herskowitz. "For example, if the harasser keeps asking you out, don't say 'Maybe another time.' " This is important, because if you later decide to file sexual harassment charges, your behavior will also be examined to determine whether the conduct was, in fact, unwanted.

In its brochure, "Sexual Harassment: It's Against the Law," the ANA recommends taking three steps in addition to confronting the harasser.[6] One, report the conduct to your supervisor, or to a higher authority if your supervisor is the harasser. If your employer has a complaint procedure, follow it; if not, take your complaint to a personnel officer.

Also, document the harassment. Write down what happened, when, how you responded, and who was there. Consider sending a certified, return-receipt letter to the harasser asking that the conduct stop. Keep a copy for yourself.

Sexual harassment: A case example

Nurse Della Saville had been an RN for more than 10 years when she enrolled in a nurse anesthetist program affiliated with a medical center in Alabama. On several occasions, her supervising instructor, CRNA Michael Shanks, allegedly made sexually suggestive comments to her. One day while working in the postop recovery room, Shanks allegedly grabbed her buttocks. When she protested, he did it a second time, and she struck him across the chest.

Saville says she confronted Shanks shortly afterwards, telling him how offended she was by his actions. He reportedly told her, according to the U.S. district court opinion, that she was "in trouble in her clinical work."

Saville reported the incident to the head of the program. Although Shanks claimed that he was just joking around when he touched Saville and that he had only touched her thigh, his supervisor warned him that he'd be fired if anything similar happened again. Shanks was also counseled about his behavior by a doctor who had witnessed the incident, and was given a written warning.

Saville agreed that Shanks was a "perfect gentlemen" to her after that. However, Shanks continued to supervise and evaluate Saville, and her clinical evaluations became increasingly negative. She was eventually dismissed from the CRNA program, allegedly because of poor performance. She filed charges

Finally, seek support from a friend, colleague, or organized group such as your state nurses association. Besides helping you emotionally, you may also learn of others who have been harassed by the same person.

And what if the harasser is a patient? Margaret Davino, RN, JD, vice president of legal affairs at St. Vincent's Hospital in New York City, advises you to tell the patient that the conduct is inappropriate and unwanted. But also inform other nurses and your supervisor, who may well be encountering the same conduct and can reinforce your message if necessary.

with the EEOC and a lawsuit against the medical center.

The facility sought summary judgment from a federal district court. But the court found enough evidence to merit a jury trial on Saville's claim that she was a victim of both quid pro quo and hostile environment sexual harassment. A jury could conclude, the court held, that her poor evaluations and ultimate discharge resulted from her refusal to acquiesce to her supervisor's alleged sexual innuendo and touching.

The court also rejected the medical center's contention that it should not be held liable because it had acted swiftly and effectively when it became aware of the harassment. The institution continued to require Saville to work under and be evaluated by Shanks, noted the court; it would be reasonable for a jury to conclude that if a hostile environment did exist, it didn't suddenly disappear just because the harassing behavior stopped.

But the jury didn't reach that conclusion. It found for Saville on her claim of quid pro quo harassment only, awarding her $150,000 in compensatory and punitive damages. The jury didn't go along with Saville's claim of wrongful discharge, finding that her poor clinical evaluations were not the result of retaliatory conduct but rather genuine performance problems unrelated to the sexual harassment.

REFERENCE
1. Saville v. Houston County Healthcare Authority, 852 F. Supp. 1512 (M.D. Ala. 1994).

Inform the patient's doctor, too, recommends Davino: "Sexual harassment should not be tolerated by any member of the patient's health care team, including the physician."

What is the employer's responsibility?

According to EEOC guidelines,[7] employers are liable for sexual harassment by supervisory personnel, regardless of whether the employer knew of the harassment.

Recently, however, some courts have ruled that employers who have clear sexual harassment reporting policies in place are not legally responsible for what happened before the harassed person registered a complaint. In other words, victims who delay reporting may be forfeiting their right to compensatory and punitive damages from the employer.

Employers are liable for the actions of a co-worker only if they knew or should have known about the harassment and failed to take immediate and effective corrective action.[7]

Any remedial action should be commensurate with the conduct, and may include a reprimand, denial of a promotion or raise, mandatory counseling, a demotion or transfer, or termination.

To prevent sexual harassment from occurring in the first place, experts say employers should have written policies on sexual harassment, including specific reporting procedures. Employees should be made aware of these policies and procedures, ideally at orientation. Indeed, some states have laws mandating the education of employees about sexual harassment.

Employers should investigate allegations of sexual harassment promptly and discretely. Be aware, however, that the accused needs to be notified of the complaint and given the opportunity to enter evidence on his behalf. That means your identity will probably be revealed to the harasser.

If the situation isn't resolved to your satisfaction, you can file a complaint with the EEOC—this generally has to be done within 180 days of the incident—and the Commission will investigate your charges. If your workplace has fewer than 15 employees, you can file a complaint with the state agency that handles discrimination cases.

Rooting out sexual harassment in the workplace isn't just one person's fight. It's the job of employees, employers, legislators, government agencies, and the courts. And that's an alliance that should make any harasser think twice.

REFERENCES

1. Equal Employment Opportunity Commission. (1995). [Sexual Harassment Statistics, 1990 – 1995].

2. Sexually harassed. (1995). Hospitals & Health Networks, 69(2), 54.

3. Childers-Hermann, J. (1993). Sexual harassment of critical care nurses. From NTI Research Abstracts. American Journal of Critical Care, 2(3), 260.

4. Libbus, M. K., & Bowman, K. G. (1994). Sexual harassment of female registered nurses in hospitals. JONA, 24(6), 26.

5. Harris v. Forklift Systems, Inc. 114 S.Ct. 367 (1993).

6. American Nurses Association. (1993). Sexual harassment: It's against the law (Item WP-3). Washington, DC: Author.

7. Equal Employment Opportunity Commission. Guidelines on discrimination because of sex. 45 FR 74677, Nov. 10, 1980.

Fighting age discrimination on the job

The experience of two RNs forced out of their jobs because of their age serves as a review of your rights under federal law.

I n recent years, employees have won many battles in the continuing fight against workplace discrimination: A Supreme Court decision in 1993 made it easier to prove sexual harassment.[1] The Americans with Disabilities Act (ADA), passed in 1990, requires employers to extend their efforts to accommodate disabled Americans. And the Age Discrimination in Employment Act of 1967 (ADEA), which went into effect in 1994, covers those who work in academia— including all RNs employed in nursing schools.

But there's a flip side to this positive picture. The wave of cost-cutting and down-sizing that's swept the nation over the last half decade appears to have given rise to an increase in age discrimination. Employers can save money by replacing highly paid senior staff with younger employees who work for less and whose health insurance coverage costs less. Increasingly, employers are choosing to do that. A case that made headlines makes it clear that RNs are not immune.

Nurses eased out after 25 years on the job

Mary Shughrue, 60, and Colleen Hoppe, 59, had worked at Sharp Memorial Hospital in San Diego for nearly 30 years. Both were exemplary employees. Shughrue did a particularly outstanding job, earning numerous merit increases in addition to her standard yearly raises. In 1989, the two nurses and a number of their colleagues were told they had to participate in a career advancement program to upgrade their job classifications to clinical nurse II. Ironically, both Shughrue and Hoppe had been working at this level for many years, even though they held the position of clinical nurse I.

Even so, both began the mandated program. They soon complained, however, that the administration was making it difficult for them to meet the new standards. Hoppe, for example, was assigned a preceptor, but later claimed that the nurse had never helped her fulfill the requirements. Shughrue reported subtle harassment: Often she would be given assignments, then have them abruptly switched for no apparent reason.

Unnerved, Shughrue decided to resign. Hoppe was ordered to resign for failing to meet the new requirements. When she flatly refused, her nurse manager fired her on the spot.[2] But the story doesn't end there: Hoppe and Shughrue fought back. Together they hired an attorney and filed a claim against Sharp Memorial for violating California's Fair Employment & Housing Act.

The part of that law that pertains to age discrimination corresponds to the federal ADEA, which protects employees aged 40 or older from being fired or denied a job, promotion, pay, or fringe benefits solely on the basis of their age. Over the years, ADEA has been bolstered by several revisions.

First, in 1987, Congress eliminated the age ceiling. Then, in 1991, the two-year statute of limitations on bringing age discrimination suits against employers was abolished, giving employees a greater opportunity to seek redress. Finally, as of December 31, 1993, ADEA applies to all employees at work sites with a staff of 20 or more.

An arbitrator rules in the nurses' favor

In January 1993, Sharp Memorial lost the case as a result of binding arbitration. The arbitrator ruled that Shughrue and Hoppe had been eased out because of their age—not, as the hospital contended, because they hadn't maintained their clinical skills. Finding the RNs "struck down and pushed out" without cause, the arbitrator ordered Sharp Memorial to pay them a total of $242,000 in damages.[2] Both nurses are currently working successfully in other positions.

Shughrue and Hoppe are just two of a steadily increasing number of employees charging age discrimination: The number of cases filed with the federal government each year is approaching 20,000, up from 15,000 in 1989. And, with courts more inclined to award punitive damages, judgments won by plaintiffs have soared, going from $30 million to $100 million in just three years time.[3] Even though nurses have filed few of these claims, many are subjected to subtle forms of age discrimination.

How ADEA fights age discrimination

Theoretically, the Age Discrimination in Employment Act is an ironclad safeguard: It not only bars unfair treatment in hiring and firing, it also declares it unlawful to "limit, segregate, or classify" employees over age 40 in a way that would deprive them of job opportunities or "adversely affect" their status as employees.[4] That makes it illegal for hospital administrators to shunt older nurses into dead-end jobs, for example, as a way of easing them out. The law also prohibits employers from giving fewer health benefits to staffers who are 65 or older than they give to other workers. Nor can nurse recruiters or other prospective employers ask a job applicant her age. Still, having these rights does not necessarily mean they are respected.

Even if you suspect you're a victim of age discrimination, though, it's tough to prove you've been wronged. Interviewers are far more likely to suggest you're overqualified than to say you're too old for a particular job. Employees who are dismissed are apt to be told it's because of institutional reorganization or their failure to master new skills—never because of age. If pressed, employers are likely to fall back on their right to hire and fire workers at will in order to justify their action. And, of course, there are often compelling—and legitimate—reasons for letting staff go. So, before concluding that you have been the object of age discrimination, it's important that you get the facts straight.

When to contact the EEOC

If you strongly believe that your employer has treated you unfairly because of your age, your first response should be to notify your supervisor, employee relations office, or personnel office. If you belong to a union, contact the representative of your local as well.

To make a strong case, you will have to show that your employer treated you—or others in your age group—differently from younger employees. To do that, you'll need to keep and submit records of incidents that point to age discrimination. You'll need to show, too, that you were fully qualified for the position you lost.

If you were dismissed from a job, find out if other older employees were also dismissed, and the reasons they were given. Look for patterns and for explanations that don't hold up. If you weren't dismissed, but have been subjected to what you believe is age discrimination, resist the urge to resign: You'll lose your rights under ADEA once you have terminated your employment.[5]

If you were denied a position or a promotion, find out who got the job. If the individual is younger than you, try to determine whether he or she has equal or better qualifications. Find out, too, if the employer has regularly turned down other older applicants and hired younger ones.

If your inquiries turn up evidence of discrimination, but your employer doesn't respond satisfactorily, you can turn to the federal government for help. You can file a report with the Equal Employment Opportunity Commission (EEOC), the federal agency responsible for eliminating discrimination in the workplace. The EEOC operates 50 field offices around the country. To get the address and telephone number of the office nearest you, call (800) 669-EEOC.

An EEOC representative will ask you to fill out a standard form describing the age discrimination you encountered and the circumstances surrounding it. Your identity will be kept confidential, at least initially. Even if your name is later revealed, ADEA prohibits employers from retaliating against an individual who files charges.

If the EEOC believes your claim may have merit, one of its representatives will notify the employer and launch an investigation of the charges.

If there's evidence substantiating your claim of age discrimination, the EEOC will attempt to work out a settlement between you and the employer. You may be offered the position you would have held if the discrimination hadn't occurred, for instance. If mediation fails—usually because the employer denies the accusation and refuses to take any corrective steps— the EEOC may press charges. In the event of litigation, the employer would have to prove that you were fired for legitimate reasons.[6]

If the EEOC does not provide the redress you're seeking, you can still file a private claim, as the California nurses did. To do so, however, you must wait at least 60 days from the time you initially filed your age discrimination complaint. If you win a private suit, the employer's penalties could include paying damages, your attorney's fees, and court costs. An employer who loses an age discrimination case is also required to post a notice promising full compliance with the law in the future.

To preserve your right to bring a private suit, however, you must bring charges of age discrimination to the EEOC within 180 days of the alleged violation; states with their own age discrimination laws have extended this deadline to 300 days, or 30 days after the termination of the EEOC's legal proceedings, whichever occurs earlier.

Age discrimination in the workplace is an insidious problem that can befall any older employee, nurses included. The best weapons you have to combat it are a clear awareness of your rights under ADEA and a willingness to fight for them when they've been threatened.

REFERENCES

1. Harris v. Forklift Systems, Inc. 510 U.S. ___ (1993).
2. Callahan, B. (1993, February 27). Sharp must pay 2 nurses $242,000. San Diego Union-Tribune, p. B2.
3. Lueck, T. J. (1993, December 12). Job-loss anger: Age bias cases soar in region. The New York Times, pp. A1, A50.
4. 29 United States Code Annotated, Sec. 623.
5. Staff. (1993). Age discrimination act violation charged: "Constructive discharge." Regan Report on Nursing Law, 34(2), 4.
6. Dowler v. New York C. & St. L. R. Co., 118 N.E. (Ill), 608; and Horsley, J. (1970). Illinois civil practice & procedure. Indianapolis: The Allen Smith Co.

Your rights when you're disabled— and afterward

The Americans with Disabilities Act extends broad protection to all employees. Here's what you should expect from your employer, or future employer, if you face discrimination because of a disability.

After an on-the-job back injury and a year out recuperating, an orthopedic charge nurse returns to work. But because her old position has been filled and she's restricted to light duty for the next few months, she's reassigned to another unit. Within eight weeks, she's fired.

Hospital officials learn from a newspaper article that a surgical tech on staff is HIV-positive. They immediately transfer him to a nonclinical job in the purchasing department.

A nurse applying for an ICU position reveals that she's a recovering drug addict. She later learns that because of her addiction, she won't be hired for the ICU slot—or for any other staff position.

Each of the health care workers in these scenarios sought legal recourse. The charge: discrimination based on a handicap. The outcomes of these cases, detailed below, highlight your rights—and the type of protection you're not entitled to—if you have a disability or incur one.

If you're qualified, employers can't just turn away

The Americans with Disabilities Act (ADA) prohibits discrimination, on the job in places of public accommodation, on the basis of a disability. The law applies specifically to any physical or mental impairment that substantially limits at least one major life activity;[1] a Senate report submitted with the act cites orthopedic, visual, and hearing deficits, multiple sclerosis, depression, HIV infection, and addiction to alcohol or drugs, among other examples.[2] Only recovering drug addicts—not current users— are protected by the ADA, though.

Employers with at least 25 workers have had to comply with the ADA since 1992. In 1994, compliance also became mandatory for businesses with 15 or more employees.

Nurses employed by facilities that get Medicare or other government funding have the protection of the federal Rehabilitation Act of 1973 as well.

To qualify for job protection under either law, a disabled person must be "otherwise qualified"—able to perform the essential job functions, either alone or with the help of "reasonable accommodations" by the employer. And "reasonable" means any change that an employer can make without undue hardship. An organization might be obligated to remove a barrier to make an office wheelchair-accessible, for example, but not to make structural changes that would cost more than its operating budget would bear. The ADA also specifies that businesses are not required to employ an individual if his disability poses a danger to the health or safety of others.

In a discrimination suit, the disabled person must demonstrate that she can do the job in question. But the burden of proving that making the necessary accommodations would create serious problems rests with the employer.

A common nursing injury ends in job loss

Mary Tuck, RN, had worked at her Tennessee hospital for 10 years when an on-the-job back injury sidelined her. When she returned to work with "light duty" physician orders, she agreed to help colleagues with light tasks in exchange for their time spent assisting her. But because Tuck could not do any lifting or pushing, an administrator fired her, contending she was unable to perform the expected duties of a staff nurse.

A trial court, and later an appeals court, disagreed, finding Tuck qualified to work as an RN. She could have performed the essential duties of the job, the appeals court found, provided reasonable accommodation—restructuring her duties or giving her a part-time or modified work schedule, for example—had been made.[3]

The court ruled that the hospital hadn't made a reasonable attempt to accommodate its employee. At the time she was fired, in fact, the hospital was advertising for nurses but didn't offer her a position.

Although the hospital contended other nurses had complained that Tuck wasn't helping them with light tasks, no written complaints had been made.

The court ordered the hospital to pay damages of nearly $27,000 and Tuck's legal expenses—and to reinstate her.

When the disability is a deadly disease

When a surgical technician at the University of Texas M.D. Anderson Cancer Center was reassigned from his clinical job because of his HIV status, he promptly sought legal recourse. The central issue facing the court was the risk of transmission of his disease to his patients.

The technician assisted in invasive procedures—work that often required his hands to be inside body cavities, in close proximity to sharp instruments—and admitted to suffering accidental puncture wounds. While the likelihood that a patient would become infected was small, the court ruled, it was not small enough "to nullify the catastrophic consequences of an accident."[4]

The only way to eliminate the risk, the court found, would be to stop the tech from doing hands-on surgical work—the essential function of his job. Thus it upheld the hospital's decision to transfer him from his OR position.

Be aware, though, that other court cases alleging discrimination against an HIV-infected health-care worker have been won by the employee. This issue continues to be decided on a case-by-case basis.

Prospective employers can't discriminate either

An RN with extensive experience in critical care answered an ad for an ICU position at a VA hospital in Wichita, Kansas. In the course of her interview, she revealed that she was a recovering drug addict, had entered a rehab program 11 months before, and was enrolled in a peer assistance program. She presented a letter of recommendation from her physician, suggesting that her access to narcotics be restricted.

Despite the RN's otherwise impressive qualifications, hospital personnel informed her that they would consider her only for a clerical job. Not being able to give narcotics, she was told, prevented her from performing the full range of an RN's duties. The court that heard the nurse's discrimination case disagreed.[5]

Giving narcotics was not an essential function of the position being applied for, the court held, and it wasn't essential that every nurse be able to do so. Reasonable accommodations like job sharing or controlled patient assignments could have allowed the RN to work in the ICU without compromising patient care.

The court also noted that the hospital had used both LPNs and graduate nurses in its ICU, even though their duties were restricted—without any evidence that doing so had jeopardized patients.

Thus it awarded the nurse back pay, benefits, and attorney's fees, and ordered the VA hospital to offer her the next available RN position.

In this case, testimony that narcotics administration comprised only 2% of an ICU nurse's time helped sway the court. But the percentage of time devoted to a particular task isn't necessarily the overriding consideration. For example, an ED nurse may not be called upon to administer narcotics frequently either. But as a member of a close-knit team that must function swiftly, her ability to do so might be considered an essential element of the job.

Where to turn if you need protection

If you think you're the victim of discrimination because of a disability, there are several places that can help. Contact the local office of the Equal Opportunity Employment Commission (EEOC), your state nurses' association, or, if necessary, an employment lawyer. If you are a member of a collective bargaining unit, talk to your union representative; doing so may result in your case being settled by arbitration, eliminating the need for litigation. Whether you are in a union or not, check your employee handbook to find out your hospital's grievance procedures.

You can also speak with someone from your human resources department and ask for information about state agencies that might be able to help. State statutes that prohibit discrimination against the disabled vary, but some may be more stringent than federal law.

If you have completed or are undergoing treatment for drug addiction or alcoholism, find out if your institution offers an employee assistance program. If it does, consider taking advantage of it; doing so may afford you extra job protection.

If you are a supervisor, examine your hospital's policies and procedures for documenting both problems with and complaints against employees. Be sure that you can support a disabled employee's termination with solid facts and documentation, should the need arise. In the Tuck case, for example, the lack of written records of problems in her new position created the impression that she was dismissed solely because of her temporary disability.

The courts have made clear that you can't be denied a job because you are unable to perform every aspect of it. The federal laws protecting the rights of the disabled to work recognize a job is often much more than the sum of its parts.

REFERENCES

1. Americans with Disabilities Act of 1990, Pub. L. 101-336, 104 Stat. 327.
2. S. Rep. No. 116, 101st Cong., 2d Sess. 22 (1990).
3. Tuck v. HCA Health Services of Tennessee, Inc., 7 F.3d 465 (6th Cir. 1993).
4. Bradley v. University of Texas M.D. Anderson Cancer Center, 3 F3d 922 (5th Cir. 1993).
5. Wallace v. Veterans Administration Medical Center, 683 F. Supp. 758 (D. Kansas, 1988).

Family leave helps you balance all your responsibilities

Who's entitled to time off and who's not?
What about contract nurses? Do you have to take
leave all at once? Here are the answers.

The federal Family and Medical Leave Act (FMLA) went into effect in 1993. In most cases it assures that you will still have a job waiting for you when you take time off in any of three situations: to care for a child after birth, adoption, or foster care placement, to care for a family member who has a serious health condition, or to deal with a serious health condition of your own that makes you unable to perform your job.

Definitions of terms under the law give you broad leeway in some areas and set strict limits in others. A serious health condition, for instance, can be anything that requires either inpatient care or continuing treatment by a health care provider. Examples include MI or CAD severe enough to require bypass surgery, stroke, back conditions requiring either extensive therapy or surgery, spinal injuries, pneumonia, severe arthritis or nervous disorders, Alzheimer's disease, and clinical depression.[1] The definition of "family members," however, includes only a spouse, parents, and children—including foster children and stepchildren. Unmarried domestic partners are excluded, as are grandparents, in-laws, and other relatives, even if they live with you.[2]

The length of time you're entitled to varies. Employers are required to grant everyone up to 12 "workweeks" of leave during a 12-month period. But the length of a workweek is determined by the number of hours you work in an average week. Thus, a nurse working 40 hours a week would be entitled to 12 40-hour workweeks of leave, for a total of 480 hours. A nurse averaging just 24 hours a week would be eligible for only 12 24-hour workweeks.

You needn't take that time all at once. Leave may be taken intermittently—a day or even an hour here and there—for doctor's appointments, for instance, or treatments. Or you can use your allotted hours to return to work part time. There is one catch, though: FMLA gives employers the right to transfer anyone who is on intermittent leave to a different but equivalent position where his or her recurrent absences would be less disruptive.

Your employer may also require you to use any or all accrued, paid leave that you are entitled to under your benefit package, collective bargaining agreement, or state disability laws as part of your 12-week allotment.

Not everyone is covered under the law

FMLA covers most federal, state, and local government employees, as well as those working for private employers. However, nurses who work in the smallest hospitals or outside of acute care should be aware that employers with fewer than 50 employees—a count that includes every staffer, full or part time, working within a 75-mile radius of the primary work site—do not have to comply with the law.

To be eligible for family leave, you must have worked for your current employer for at least 12 months and put in a minimum of 1,250 hours during the 12 months immediately preceding the start of your leave. Since independent contractors are not covered, per diem and other contract nurses should review the terms of their employment carefully to find out if they qualify.

Giving notice, getting documentation

If you anticipate taking leave, you must give your employer 30 days' notice, verbally or in writing. If your leave is unforeseeable, or has to begin sooner than planned—because of premature labor, for example—you must notify your employer as soon as possible. When leave is prompted by medical problems, your employer can require a written statement from your health care provider, justifying your request. FMLA allows your employer to request certification from a second provider, this one of his choice, if he's not satisfied with the initial explanation. And if the two opinions differ, a third—and deciding—opinion may be sought from a clinician both parties agree on.

FMLA recognizes advanced practice nurses: Certified nurse-midwives and nurse practitioners are among the health care providers authorized to provide such certification.

FMLA, job security, and fringe benefits

If you take family leave, are you guaranteed you'll get your job back? Generally, the answer is Yes. In fact, the law makes it illegal for your employer to discourage you or interfere when you seek to take leave. And you can't be fired for taking an authorized leave. When you return from leave, however, your employer can change your position, provided the one you're offered is equivalent—in seniority, status, salary, benefits, working conditions, and other terms—to what you enjoyed before. The law entitles you to a job on the same shift and with the same, or an equivalent, work schedule as well.

Ironically, the more powerful your position, the more problems you're apt to face: FMLA does not guarantee job security to nurses in top management. A "key employee"—one whose earnings rank in the organization's top 10%—may be denied reinstatement. But the employer can't spring this on a staff member by surprise: She must receive written notice of her "key employee" status under the law when she requests leave, and her employer must prove that restoring her to the position would cause the organization "substantial and grievous economic injury."[1]

While you're on leave, your employer must continue to provide health benefits under the same terms in effect when you work. Thus, you're responsible for any premiums, including increases, that you'd normally pay. If you plan to take extended unpaid leave, check with your benefits coordinator to be sure you'll have uninterrupted coverage.

If you decide not to return to your job—to stay home with your baby or to relocate, for instance—you will have to reimburse your employer for any health or other benefits paid for while you were on leave. Reimbursement won't be necessary if your own ill health or that of a family member prevents your return.

Although FMLA is effective in all 50 states and in the District of Columbia, it does not replace any state law that's more generous. Instead, it sets minimum rights that cannot be reduced under state law, collective bargaining agreement, or employer policy. Terms of employment or state disability, maternity, or family leave laws may provide additional or different benefits, however, which must be coordinated with your rights under FMLA.

For example, under District of Columbia law a nurse may be eligible for up to 16 workweeks of personal medical leave and up to 16 workweeks of family care leave over a two-year period, so it's possible that a nurse could use her entire 32 weeks of leave in one year and still be eligible for 12 weeks of federal leave the following year. District law considers domestic partners family members as well.[3]

If you have any questions about how much or what type of leave you're entitled to, consult a knowledgeable benefits manager, union representative, state or federal agency, or an attorney.

The FMLA requires employers to post notice of employee rights and provide detailed information upon request. Should a legal dispute arise about your rights under the law or if you feel your rights have been violated, contact your local branch of the Department of Labor, Wage and Hour Division.

Under certain circumstances, you can file a civil lawsuit against your employer for violation of the law. You may seek reinstatement to your job and compensatory damages for lost wages, benefits, and other costs, such as wages paid to a home health nurse or sitter when leave was improperly denied.

The Family and Medical Leave Act does not solve all dilemmas arising from the conflict between your own needs or those of a family member and the demands of your job. And it does come with some strings attached. But the law goes a long way in helping employees cope with one kind of crisis without having to worry about facing another.

REFERENCES

1. Senate Committee Report on the Family and Medical Leave Act, #103-3A, Jan. 27, 1993.
2. The Family and Medical Leave Act of 1993, P.L. 103-3, and 29 CFR Part 825.
3. Section 36-1301 et.seq. D.C. Code, Annotated, 1981.

If you're fired

Learn your rights if you lose your job—
and those you have when
looking for another—with this "case study."

Heather Goldberg, RN, arrived at her attorney's office confused, hurt, and uncertain. She had just been dismissed from the hospital job that she had held for 15 years. Without notice, severance pay, or even a reason.

She said her employer had been in the throes of "redesigning," but she had no idea that someone with her seniority and skills would be let go. She wanted to know if her termination was legal, what benefits she's entitled to, and her rights when she applies for a new job.

With downsizing and re-engineering no longer a rarity in health care, it pays to know what protections the law affords you.

The risks of working without a contract

Heather, like most nurses, was an at-will employee. She had no employment contract and was not covered by a collective bargaining agreement. Nurses who belong to a union may have several weeks notice of their termination, and possibly a severance package.

At-will employment offers no such guarantees: Both employer and employee can generally terminate the working relationship whenever they like, without giving notice or a reason. Courts have recognized the disparity in bargaining power between employee and employer, though, and have developed some exceptions to the rule of at-will termination.

First, the employer must act in good faith. A dismissal based on fabricated charges or motivated by a personal grudge, for example, may be found illegal. Even "inexplicable" terminations—where there is no apparent reason for firing the employee—are subject to the scrutiny of the courts.

Second, employees cannot be fired for reasons inconsistent with public policy. Terminations that have been deemed to violate public policy include ones carried out in retaliation for performing an important and socially desirable act, such as serving on a jury; exercising a statutory right, such as filing a workers' compensation claim; or refusing to commit an unlawful act, such as perjury.

The public policy exception applies whether you work in a public or private hospital and regardless of what reason the employer may actually choose to give you.

Many states also have "whistle-blower" statutes. They are designed to protect employees who report what they have reasonable cause to believe are illegal acts by their employer.

Be aware that while courts in some states tend to be "pro-employee," those in others interpret the doctrine of at-will employment strictly and are less inclined to recognize exceptions. To find out what specific legal protections exist for employees in your state, a good place to start is the local library.

None of the exceptions to at-will termination seemed to apply in Heather's case, but her hospital's policy and procedure manual might offer help, particularly the sections describing termination procedures. These documents may create an employment contract, modifying the employee's at-will status.

For example, the procedures for termination may require progressive disciplinary measures or written notice before firing. However, even if the employer violates its own procedures, the employee may still not be able to successfully sue for wrongful discharge. That's because courts do not always view these manuals as enforceable contracts.

To make that all but certain, many employers include disclaimers in their manuals stating that the contents are not conditions of employment and are not binding. That was the case with the manual Heather showed her lawyer, leaving them no grounds for proceeding against the hospital on that basis.

But some other information Heather gave the lawyer raised a red flag: Her pension was due to be fully vested in a few months, she is nearly 52 years old, and a nurse who was fired at the same time is also in her 50s.

The attorney told Heather they could seriously look into the possibility that she had been targeted because of her age. The Age Discrimination in Employment Act (ADEA) protects employees 45 and older from being fired solely on the basis of age. Other federal legislation protects workers of all ages from job actions based on sex, race, national origin, religion, color, pregnancy, or disability.

There's also the possibility that Heather's discharge violated the Employment Retirement Income Security Act (ERISA). This act makes it illegal to fire an employee to prevent pension benefits from vesting.

Before proceeding, her attorney advised Heather to write to the hospital's human resource department requesting a written reason for her dismissal. A reply could prove valuable—if she decides to contest her termination, for example, or if her employer challenges her right to collect unemployment. Some states even require employers to comply with such requests. You can contact your state labor department to see if yours does.

Are you qualified for unemployment benefits?

Since investigating the possibility of age discrimination and an ERISA violation would take time, the attorney advised Heather not to put her life on hold—she should start looking for work and making financial arrangements for the interim.

Heather is eligible for unemployment. Not all terminated employees are: A willful and wanton disregard for the employer's interests, such as theft of a patient's belongings, consistent poor work attendance, and resignation—even one submitted because the employer changed your working conditions—have all been grounds for denial of benefits.

There are certain cases, however, in which a person who resigns will still qualify for unemployment benefits. Resignation prompted by continued sexual harassment is one of them.

Her unemployment check will provide Heather with up to two-thirds of her former salary, although states set a dollar limit that may be much lower than that level. Benefits usually continue for up to 26 weeks, but the state can extend or shorten this period.

To collect, Heather has to search for a job and may be asked to prove it—by supplying the names of places she has applied to, for example. But she doesn't have to accept a job offer if the position pays substantially less than her previous one, is in a different specialty, or would present a significant hardship, such as requiring a live-in sitter while she worked nights.

Fortunately for Heather, her hospital has a written policy of reimbursing employees for unused vacation time—a week in her case. Employers who do not have such policies may not be required to do so.

Like all employers, Heather's hospital is required by the Consolidated Omnibus Budget Reconciliation Act (COBRA) to give her the option of continuing her health insurance for up to 18 months once her policy lapses, which is usually a month or so after employment ends. She'll have to pay the premium the hospital had been paying for her, though, which is likely to be hefty.

Job applicants have protections, too

With fewer nursing positions available and employers who are able to be very selective, Heather is afraid she won't be hired because of her age. Nurses who have a disability or belong to a minority group may also worry about their chances of getting a new job.

Fortunately, the Americans with Disabilities Act (ADA) has made it easier for disabled individuals to get a fair shake: The law prohibits employers from asking questions about disabilities on job application forms and in interviews. Federal and state anti-discrimination laws have also largely eliminated questions about age, past medical history, health, workers' compensation claims, pregnancy, race, national origin, religion, and gender.

Employers can elicit such information only if it directly relates to the "essential functions" of the job. And the questions must be phrased in a way that reflects that. For example, the interviewer can't ask if you have a disability, or the extent or nature of it if it's apparent. But you may be asked about your ability to lift patients or perform other nursing tasks.

If you have a disability but the employer can provide reasonable accommodations for it, you can't be denied a job solely on the basis of your handicap.

Heather, like all job applicants, can be required to take a pre-employment test as long as it is strictly job-related and consistent with business necessity, such as an exam on medications that nurses administer.

Employers have the right to screen applicants for illegal drug use, too. They can also require a medical exam, but only after a conditional job offer has been made. The tests and exam must be a usual part of the hiring process and be administered to all prospective employees in the same job category.

Employers can reject a candidate if the drug test is positive or the medical exam reveals a condition that would preclude the candidate from performing one of the job's essential functions. But, whether you're hired or not, employers must keep exam results confidential; only those who need to know—such as your prospective supervisor—can be told.

The next few weeks or months will not be easy for Heather, but they don't have to be overwhelming either. Armed with information about her rights, and with the names of a job counselor and placement agency in hand, she left her attorney's office ready to begin a new phase in her career.

Q&A:
Rights and
Responsibilities

Workers' comp for this illness?

*I work in a brand new facility, and was recently hospitalized and
diagnosed with sick building syndrome. Do I have any legal recourse?*
Sick building syndrome is believed to occur because of an accumulation of contaminants in a new building and the subsequent
reduction in the supply of fresh air. Its manifestations include
irritation of the eyes, nose, throat, and skin, headache, fatigue,
difficulty concentrating, diarrhea, and asthma-like symptoms.

Employees who develop health problems that are the result of
occupational exposure to indoor air pollution typically file workers'
compensation claims. So, if your condition is preventing you
from returning to your place of employment, you can apply for
workers' comp.

There is no guarantee, however, that your compensation
claim will be approved. Assessing disability in workers who are
suspected of having sick building syndrome is difficult because
there is usually no evidence of any type of permanent impairment.
What's more, some physicians dispute that the syndrome
even exists. And, its manifestations are so nonspecific that a
diagnosis isn't usually made unless many workers in the
building are afflicted.

If you do receive workers' compensation, the law precludes
you from suing your employer for damages. However, you may
be able to file a suit against a third party, such as the construction
company, if they violated state or federal laws governing the
quality of indoor air.

Manditory TB testing: your choice?

*My employer is requiring nurses to have an annual tuberculosis test. Is it
legal to mandate such testing and can I be suspended if I don't comply?*
With the re-emergence of tuberculosis, private hospitals are now
mandated by OSHA to establish TB exposure control programs.
Public health care institutions generally adhere to this mandate,

as well. One component of the program is annual skin testing of hospital personnel, even those who are not directly involved with patient care.

Perhaps with the hospital's permission you could undergo an annual chest X-ray instead of the skin test. But if this isn't an option and you still refuse to be tested, the hospital could fire you for not complying with its rules and regulations and for posing a danger to patients.

Work-related injuries off the job

During a winter storm I was called into work because we were short-staffed. On the way in, I got in a car accident. Are my injuries covered by workers' comp?

Generally, employees are not considered to be operating within the scope of their employment on the way to and from work and are therefore ineligible under workers' comp for injuries incurred at those times. There are exceptions, however, in instances where there is a clear connection between the employment and the risk to the employee.

A case in point: An RN who worked overtime because she couldn't find a replacement for a sick employee, as required by hospital policy, fell asleep on her drive home and crashed into a pole. She filed a workers' comp claim for her injuries and the workers' compensation board upheld it. She'd fallen asleep, the board members concluded, as a direct result of the unusually long hours she'd been required to work—28 out of 40. Under those circumstances, the board declared, the accident was a "reasonably anticipated hazard."

The same sort of exception might be made in your case. Contact the human resources office or benefits counselor at work and, if necessary, your local workers' compensation office. If you still have questions regarding your eligibility for coverage, consult a lawyer who specializes in workers' comp cases.

Advocacy for patients vs. job security

As an RN working in a nursing home, I'm obligated to report abuse and neglect of my patients. But as an "at will" employee, I'm concerned about reprisals—including being fired—if I do. How can I protect both my patients and my job?

There is no magic answer. Most states mandate by statute that you report suspected abuse or neglect of elderly patients to the appropriate state agency. Your professional code as a nurse compels you to speak up, too. In the real world, though, where most employees can be fired at their employer's discretion, reporting may well have repercussions for you.

If you were to be fired, though, you may have grounds for a lawsuit if the dismissal violated public policy—in this case, protection of patients' health and safety. The public policy exception to at-will employment is supposed to uphold policies that exist for the public good. For example, courts have upheld lawsuits where employees have been fired in retaliation for reporting employers' violations of OSHA rules and the Civil Rights Act.

Unfortunately, it's not always clear if and when the public policy exception applies; the courts make this determination based on case and statutory law, and some states are more favorable to employees than others. If your state has a whistle-blower statute, this may afford you added protection.

For now, the best strategy is to be prepared to defend yourself in the event you are fired. Follow your facility's reporting policy on what and where to document suspected abuse or neglect. Often, this will trigger an internal investigation but if not, take your concerns up the chain of command. Keep a copy of all memos you send. If the problem remains unresolved, report it to the appropriate state agency as required by law.

Having a baby shouldn't hurt your job status

*I'm about to return to work from maternity leave and just found out
I've been reassigned to a lower-level position on another unit. My
supervisor attributes the move to "restructuring." Is that legal?*
Not if you took the leave under disability coverage offered
through your employer. The Pregnancy Discrimination Act
mandates that employers provide time off for childbirth on the
same terms as other disability leaves and restore you to the same
or equivalent position when you return.

The same holds true if you took the time off under the
Family and Medical Leave Act (FMLA)—unless your salary ranks
among the top 10% at your facility. That group of workers is not
entitled to automatic reinstatement under the federal law. The
employer does, however, have to provide the worker with written
notice of her "key employee" status when she requests her leave.

Check your employee handbook to see the terms of your
leave. Then sit down with your supervisor to review the handbook,
as well as any previous memos and conversations pertaining to
your time off. If that doesn't resolve the problem, lodge a
complaint either with your state's EEOC office or, if you took
leave under FMLA, with the local office of the U.S. Department
of Labor.

Working a second job

*I'm thinking about working part-time at another hospital to supplement
my income. Can my employer prohibit me from moonlighting?*
Unless a written restriction already exists—in the form of a
union contract or other employment agreement, for example—
you're free to work as many jobs as you like. Your employer
could make a performance issue out of your second job, however,
if, for instance, you started showing up late.

If you did agree in writing not to work for anyone else, your
employer could sue you for violating that agreement and possibly
prevent you from keeping your second job.

Often, prohibitions against second jobs are used by employers who have a hard time recruiting employees and worry about staffers being lured away by competitors. In health care, such restrictions are more likely to apply to physicians and certified nurse-midwives than to staff nurses. Just how strictly courts enforce such "noncompete" agreements, though, varies widely.

Do employee manuals have the force of law?

My hospital revised its employee handbook several years after I was hired. Am I still covered by the provisions in the manual I received when I was hired?

Not necessarily. Although an employer may be bound ethically by the provisions in an employee manual, there may not be a corresponding legal obligation. Most employers maintain that their employee handbooks are not contracts. But courts have found that whether a manual constitutes a contractual agreement often depends on what's in it. So, many hospitals steer clear of legal problems by adding disclaimers that state that the manual is not a binding agreement and can be revised at any time.

If your employer says the revised version now applies, there's probably not much you can do about it. If you have a union contract or other written employment agreement, however, you do not have to abide by any changes that violate the terms of those agreements.

Antidiscrimination laws for gays

I've been passed over for several promotions recently, and a colleague intimated that it's because of my sexual orientation. What recourse do I have?

Although federal law prohibits on-the-job discrimination based on age, gender, disability, race, or religion, there is no corresponding federal protection for gays and lesbians. A number of cities and some states do have statutes that prohibit discrimination based on sexual orientation, however.

If you live in a jurisdiction that does—and this may vary even within state lines—you can file a complaint with the appropriate administrative agency, for example, the state or city human rights' division. If you don't know whether you are protected by an antidiscrimination statute or which agency to contact, your city attorney's office or local EEOC may be able to tell you.

Even if you do have a legal basis for fighting workplace discrimination, I would advise you to try to work out this matter internally first. Meet with your supervisor to express your interest in advancement, if you haven't already done so. In a nonaccusatory manner, ask whether she thinks you're a candidate for promotion and why you did not get the previous promotions. Document the date and content of your discussion and keep it for future reference.

Select your job references with care

When a recruiter checked my references and then told me I wouldn't be hired because I wasn't "right" for the job, I figured one of them said something that changed her mind. Do I have any rights in this situation?
Under common law, employers enjoy a "qualified privilege" when sharing information about present or former employees. This privilege typically shields them from claims of libel or slander. However, certain communications—repeating recklessly inaccurate information, rumors, or personal facts that are irrelevant to the individual's ability to do the job—are not protected. If a former employer did any of these things, you may be able to sue.

To find out, try asking the recruiter to be more specific about what makes you unsuitable for the position. Check with your references to see if they were contacted and what information they gave out. Despite the qualified privilege protection, many employers still fear being sued and provide only written references or basic information.

If you fail to uncover anything, your best bet may be to rethink whom you give as a reference.

Allegations can endanger your license

I was suspended after being accused of harming a patient and rein-stated when a hospital investigation cleared me of wrongdoing. I'm concerned about repercussions. Should I be?

Yes; depending on your state's regulations, your license could be in jeopardy. An employer is obligated to report professional employees whose conduct or care endangers patients to the department of public health, state licensing board, and/or other state agency. With the exception of some criminal reporting requirements, such as suspected child abuse, this report should usually be made only after a full investigation. In reality, though, some employers jump the gun.

A patient also has the right to file a complaint against you with the appropriate state agency. So just because your employer has resolved the matter internally doesn't mean your case is closed.

You'll be notified if the board of nursing decides to investigate a complaint filed against you. If that happens, I strongly advise you to consult an attorney before filing any response to the charges.

In the meantime, insist on a copy of the allegations against you from your employer if you have not already received it and a letter stating that you have been cleared of all charges. Also, ask to see your personnel file to verify that it contains no falsely incriminating statements.

If a pregnant worker wants reassignment

I'm pregnant and because some of my patients have TB, I'm worried. If I ask to be reassigned, is my employer required to accommodate me?

No. Although pregnancy may constitute a short-term disability, it does not qualify you for protection under the Americans with Disabilities Act, which requires most employers to make reason-able accommodations for disabled employees.

The federal Pregnancy Discrimination Act prohibits discrimi-nation against pregnant employees, but does not mandate that they be given preferential treatment. So unless other employees caring for TB patients have been reassigned upon request, your employer has no compelling reason to reassign you.

An Alabama appeals court made that point recently in rejecting a discrimination claim filed by a home health nurse who was fired for refusing to care for an AIDS patient during her pregnancy. The court found that the employer had treated pregnant and nonpregnant employees equally, in accordance with the law.

When "Don't ask, don't tell" is wise

During a recent job interview, I was asked if I had any children. Is that legal? And how should I have answered it?

Merely asking whether a job applicant has children is not illegal; some interviewers use personal questions as a conversation ice breaker. However, because asking may open the door to a charge of discrimination, most interviewers wisely steer clear of the question.

You could have refused to answer the question because it is not relevant to your ability to do the job. Realistically, though, such a response may well have decreased your likelihood of getting the job. If you suspect that you did not get the position because of your reply, you can contact your local EEOC office or state civil rights commission, who may decide to investigate your complaint.

Keep in mind, though, that it may be very difficult to prove that you were not hired because of your answer or the size of your family, or that the employer's intent in asking the question was discriminatory.

Your right to be paid for overtime

I worked five hours of overtime filling in for a sick colleague recently but I have never been compensated for it. My supervisor told me that's because I failed to get formal approval before working the extra hours. Is that legal?

Under the provisions of the Fair Labor Standards Act, full-time, hourly employees who are not in management positions are usually entitled to overtime pay. But only those hours worked above and beyond a 40-hour work week are considered to be overtime.

Because your supervisor knew you were working those extra hours, she gave you her implied approval; that is sufficient for you to be compensated. Review the circumstances of the overtime in question with her, and point out that you are indeed entitled to be paid. Check for a written policy and, if necessary, take your case to your hospital's human resources department.

If you cannot resolve the matter internally, call the Department of Labor's Wage and Hour Division. The number will be listed in your local phone book.

If you're let go without a detailed reason

Just four months after starting a new position, I was fired, allegedly for making a medication error. When I asked my supervisor to elaborate, she refused. Was it legal for my employer to fire me without an adequate explanation?

It depends on the state in which you work: More than half have statutes requiring employers to give a specific and valid reason for the dismissal of a nurse or any other licensed professional. In the remaining states, nurses are employed "at will," and their employers have no such obligation.

In the case you describe, your rights may also depend on hospital policy, so check your employee handbook. For example, some employers in "at will" states nonetheless stipulate that they will provide employees who are dismissed with a valid reason.

If you haven't done so, speak with the assistant director of nursing, director of nursing, or a chief administrator. If you don't get answers, contact your state labor department to find out whether you were entitled to an explanation. If so, file a complaint with the labor department against the employer.

Whenever you start a new job it is a good idea to ask a staffer from the personnel department to detail the terms of hiring and dismissal or layoff—not an uncommon concern in this era of downsizing. Then write down whatever assurances you receive and keep this for future reference. If your employer later violates this written or verbal agreement, report it to your state's labor department.

The Legal Process

Safeguarding your license: Avoid these pitfalls

Clinical knowledge and skill aren't the only things you need to hang on to your license. Here's what you need to know to protect your right to practice.

A patient tells his nurse that his pain during the night was unbearable—why wasn't he given any medication? The nurse checks the chart; it indicates that meds were administered every three hours. Suspicious, the nurse alerts her supervisor, who investigates and concludes that the night nurse is stealing narcotics. She notifies the state licensing board, which suspends the night nurse from practice and orders her to complete a drug rehabilitation program.

A nurse taking a licensure exam answers "No" to a question asking if she has ever been arrested. She passes the exam and receives her license—only to have it revoked when the licensing board discovers that she was arrested for shoplifting 22 years before.[1] She is able to get her license back only by agreeing to write an open letter to nursing students telling them of her license revocation.

These are just a couple of the hundreds of disciplinary cases brought to attorneys over the years. Some have involved flagrant breaches of professional standards; others less severe violations. In many, the nurse wasn't even aware that she had put her license at risk.

Let's review some common ways that nurses jeopardize their licenses—and discuss what you can do to avoid endangering your own.

How nurses cross the line

Every state has an agency—commonly known as the Board of Nursing—that regulates the practice of nursing. Using the Nurse Practice Act and other state laws as its guide, the board defines the responsibilities of the nurse and grants licenses to applicants who meet its standards. Any time a nurse is charged with violating those standards, the board may conduct an investigation and, if appropriate, take disciplinary action—up to and including suspension or revocation of the nurse's license.

The reasons that nurses get into trouble are many, ranging from criminal behavior—such as forging a physician's signature—to "unprofessional conduct." This can include anything from failing to keep CPR training current to failing to sign out medications. Here's a rundown of the most common types of cases that come before the board:

Negligence. Instances in which a nurse provides substandard care or does not do her job in a reasonably prudent manner can lead to a negligence charge. A nurse can be disciplined by the board even though the failure to meet the standard of care did not result in actual injury to the patient. A nurse may be considered negligent, for example, if she administers the wrong medication and doesn't inform the physician of that fact or if she improperly delegates duties to assistive personnel.

Patient neglect is also a form of negligence. One such case involved a home health nurse who made weekly visits to a mentally retarded patient who was on medication. While the nurse was on vacation, a colleague filled in and discovered that the patient hadn't been bathed or fed and was living in extreme filth. The colleague filed a complaint with the Board of Nursing, alleging neglect. The board placed the home health nurse on probation for six months and required her to go through her employer's orientation program again.

Whether one instance of negligence is enough to cost you your license will depend on the circumstances of the case, your professional record, and the patient's condition. It's possible, though, that a single incident in an otherwise stellar career could result in the loss of your license.

Incompetence. Unlike negligence, in which a nurse is capable of rendering the necessary care but does not do it, incompetence is the charge applied to a nurse who is not qualified to provide care. The charge may be levied against experienced nurses as well as new ones.

Let's say, for instance, that you are a float nurse with no intensive care training or experience and you're given an assignment in a specialized ICU. You jeopardize not only the patients, but your license if you accept the assignment and provide care that you're not qualified to give. The fact that you shouldn't have been given the assignment in the first place won't serve as a valid defense.

Abusive behavior. This may be either verbal or physical in nature, although exactly what constitutes "abuse" may be open to interpretation. In one case, for instance, a nurse was assisting a patient from the bathroom back to the bed when the patient became disoriented and kept trying to sit on the floor. The frustrated nurse told the patient, "Move your ****ing backside."

The remark was overheard by a nurse's aide, and reported to the head nurse and, ultimately, the Board of Nursing. In its investigation, the board found that the remark rose to the level of patient abuse and placed the nurse on probation for one year.

Drug or alcohol abuse. Many state boards report chemical dependency as the number one reason for disciplinary action.[2] Sanctions often include license suspension, mandatory participation in a drug rehab program, and a probationary period in which certain practice restrictions are imposed—not being allowed to care for patients who are receiving narcotics, for instance.

Even though impaired nurses pose a great risk to patients, many boards of nursing are reluctant to revoke their licenses because they recognize that the nurse has an addiction and needs help.

Physical or mental impairment. Conditions such as loss of motor skill or mobility—be they the result of injury, organic disease, or simply growing old—render some nurses unable to provide safe care, and, therefore, may be grounds for intervention by the board. So can mental illnesses such as schizophrenia and disorders such as panic attacks.

Having a physical or mental impairment doesn't *necessarily* mean that your license is in jeopardy, though. The Americans with Disabilities Act requires your employer to provide reasonable accommodations to help you do your job safely. But, if an incident does occur and your capacity is questioned, the board may order you to submit to a mental or physical exam to determine your fitness to continue nursing.

Fraud. Deceptive acts committed while attempting to procure a nursing license, such as lying about an arrest record or academic history, are grounds for disciplinary action. So is fraud committed in the course of professional activities, such as falsifying an insurance claim form or hospital or patient records.

Take the case of a nursing supervisor at a convalescent home who failed to sign an incident report within 48 hours of a patient's fall—a policy spelled out in the facility's policies and procedures. Realizing her error, she used correction fluid to change the date of the incident to coincide with that of her signature. She also failed to forward the report to the appropriate state agency—again disregarding policy.

The nursing department reported her to the board, which placed her on probation for a year. The nursing home doled out its own punishment: It fired her.

How to safeguard your right to practice

One important way to protect your license is to know and follow the provisions of the Nurse Practice Act in the states where you work. You can obtain a copy of the act from the state Board of Nursing.

You should also be familiar with the Patient's Bill of Rights. The American Hospital Association first promulgated a model declaration in the 1970s. Hospitals have modified that as their situations dictated and most facilities give patients a copy when they're admitted. Since the patient's rights and responsibilities vary from facility to facility it's a good idea to review those in force at your work setting. Violating any of these rights could be grounds for disciplinary action as well as a malpractice suit.

Be sure to completely, accurately, and objectively document all care and teaching that you provide. Doing so can help you both avoid disciplinary action and defend against it. Read and follow your employer's policies and procedures for documenting care and teaching and for correcting errors in the patient's chart.

Always remember that your primary obligation is to protect the patient, and let that principle be your guide. You should question any order that:

- could result in undue harm to the patient,
- conflicts with the terms of your license,
- is illegal,
- goes against hospital policy, or
- you are not qualified to carry out.

Discuss your concerns with the person who gave the order; take the matter up the chain of command if necessary. Document the conversation according to your facility's policy— whether that means documenting your concerns in the patient's chart or in an incident report.

If you suspect that a colleague's conduct endangers a patient's well-being, report this to the appropriate authorities. In fact, some states mandate that you do so.

Finally, if you're working with unlicensed assistive personnel, know how and what to delegate. Although there are few if any cases in which an RN has been held accountable for the negligent acts of an unlicensed aide, improper delegation or supervision are grounds for disciplinary action.

To avoid problems, read your state's Nurse Practice Act or your facility's policies to determine which tasks can be delegated and which must be reserved for licensed nurses. Then match the right task to the right person by familiarizing yourself with the assistant's job description, background, and training. You should consider the nature and complexity of the task, along with the patient's acuity. Provide adequate supervision—an inexperienced aide or difficult task will require closer supervision—and make sure you are readily available if the unlicensed staffer needs your assistance.

Whether its delegating tasks, performing a procedure, or documenting care, know what's expected of you ahead of time. It's the best way to protect what you've worked hard to earn: the right to call yourself a practicing nurse.

REFERENCES

1. Twenty-two years is a long time. (1995, Summer). Nursing Report, 10(2), 1.
2. Fiesta, J. (1990). The impaired nurse—who is liable. Nursing Management, 21(10), 20.

Safeguarding your license: The disciplinary process

A step-by-step guide to help you through a Board of Nursing investigation.

Y ou receive a letter from the state Board of Nursing informing you that Michael Davis, a former patient, has filed a complaint alleging that you physically abused him. The board is investigating whether or not to file disciplinary charges against you.

Your mind is immediately filled with questions: What are my rights? Will there be a hearing? Can I lose my license?

No one wants to be in a position to have to ask those questions, but if you do need to defend yourself successfully before the state board, you need to know how the investigative and disciplinary processes work.

A single complaint triggers action

Anyone can file a complaint with the Board of Nursing—a patient, a colleague, a physician, or a hospital administrator. As the agency responsible for regulating the practice of nursing, the board has a duty to investigate any and all allegations and, when appropriate, to take disciplinary action.

If the board receives sufficient evidence that a nurse represents a clear and immediate danger to the public's health and safety, it can summarily revoke or suspend that nurse's license. It can do the same if it's notified that a nurse has been convicted of a violent crime or has had her license revoked in another state.

Normally, though, the nursing boards in most states afford the accused certain rights, as outlined in the due process clause of the Constitution: Before it can take any formal action against a nurse's license, it should inform her in writing of the allegations against her, the ensuing investigation, and any formal disciplinary charges that it decides to file. And it must give the nurse the opportunity to defend herself.

If you're ever notified about a complaint, the board may ask you to provide a written response to the allegations within a specified time. Be objective when phrasing your response. Avoid using subjective terms like, "I feel that the charges are unfounded." Rather, list factual information related to the event or behavior in question. If possible, list the names of witnesses who might be able to corroborate your story.

Before submitting your response, consult an attorney. Although some malpractice policies may cover attorney fees in disciplinary matters, most don't. So you'll need to retain private counsel. You should select one who has experience defending nurses before the board.

The American Association of Nurse Attorneys (TAANA), based in Ellicott City, Md., can provide you with the name of the chapter president in your area who can refer you to a nurse attorney. Although retaining counsel isn't cheap—nurse attorneys generally charge $125 – $200 an hour—it's a small price to pay to protect your livelihood.

Do not talk to anyone about the case without your attorney's approval—not your supervisor, co-workers, witnesses, or the person who made the allegation against you. If you do, you might inadvertently say something that could be used against you. Do, however, notify your liability insurance carrier if the allegation was made by a patient who was injured, since there's a good possibility that he'll file a malpractice claim against you as well.

The investigation: What to expect

Typically, investigators for the board will contact any and all witnesses for information and statements about the complaint. They will also subpoena pertinent medical records and get a copy of your facility's policies and procedures. The board may also retain an independent nurse consultant to review your nursing notes in any relevant charts and to determine if the actions you took were appropriate.

In cases where a nurse is suspected of diverting drugs for her own use or for sale, the federal Drug Enforcement Agency (DEA) may conduct an investigation of its own. It may, for instance, have an undercover agent monitor the nurse at work. The board can then use the DEA's findings as evidence against the nurse.

Once the board's investigation is complete—and assuming it's found merit in the charges—an attorney employed by the state will schedule a conference with you and, usually, your lawyer. (If your attorney isn't invited by the state, bring him or her along anyway.) At the conference, the state attorney, or a panel of board members, will review the results of the investigation and tell you what formal charges could be filed. By the end of the conference, you should have a good understanding of the evidence that will be presented if your case goes to a hearing before either the entire board or a representative panel.

Next, members of the board meet privately to review the investigators' findings and the recommendations of the state attorney or board panel to decide whether to file formal charges.

If they decide to do so, they may also choose to allow you to sign a consent agreement to save both you and the board the time and expense of going through a hearing. The consent agreement usually carries a sanction that's less severe than the penalties that could be imposed if the matter went to a hearing. For example, the board might decide to put you on probation or require you to take continuing education courses. If you choose not to accept the offer, a full hearing will be scheduled.

Defending your license before the board

It may be months before you can defend yourself at a full hearing. Some boards meet only once a month and not at all during the summer. And, when your case finally does come up, it may be held over until the next board meeting if things run late and time runs out.

In the meantime, you and your attorney will work on your defense. Your job is to provide her with complete and accurate information about the event. Be sure to describe your actions, the patient's response if applicable, your facility's policies and procedures, and the rationale behind any deviation from the standard of care.

Your attorney's job is to prepare you for the proceedings. She'll obtain statements from witnesses and pertinent data such as medical records and review these documents with you. You will be questioned about this material—as well as your own actions—if your attorney calls you to testify at the hearing. To help their clients prepare for testifying, attorneys sometimes stage mock depositions.

The hearing itself is less formal than a trial: It's held in a government facility but not a courtroom, and the parties convene around a conference table. Nonetheless, it's important to dress conservatively and be prompt; you need to look and act like the professional you are.

An attorney representing the state—usually from the attorney general's office—will present the charges and evidence from their investigation, including testimony of witnesses. Although written statements may be presented, for the most part witnesses testify in person and are then cross-examined by your attorney.

Once the state completes its case, the defense gets its chance to present witnesses and evidence. If you're called to testify, listen carefully to each question posed by your lawyer and the attorney who cross-examines you. Answer succinctly; don't provide any more information than is asked for. For example, if you're asked what medication you administered to Mr. Davis on a particular morning, say "Penicillin." Don't embellish your answer by stating what meds you administered that afternoon or the next morning.

Answer all questions out loud and audibly—the stenographer who's recording the proceedings can't transcribe a nod of your head.

Finally, members of the board may have questions of their own. Although they rarely interrupt testimony, they can ask witnesses to testify about matters that they feel have not been adequately covered.

The decision and your future

Once the hearing is over, you may or may not have a long wait before you find out your fate. Some boards decide cases on the same day as the hearing; others take months to announce a decision.

If the decision goes your way, the board will provide written notice to all parties involved that you have been cleared of any wrongdoing. Be sure to show this notice to your supervisor or employer if they were aware of the charges.

If the board decides against you, it will take one or more of the following actions:

- Censure you—state their disapproval of your actions in the minutes of one of their meetings,
- Issue a letter of reprimand—a more severe way of expressing their disapproval of your actions,
- Place you on probation—monitor your professional activities for a certain period of time,
- Suspend your license—prohibit you from practicing for a defined period, or
- Revoke your license—the most severe penalty, which prohibits you from ever practicing again.

If you disagree with the board's decision or the penalties imposed, you can file an appeal with a trial court. Keep in mind, though, that appeals can be costly and lengthy—it may take several years before the matter is finally concluded.

Hopefully, you'll never have to defend your license. But if you do, knowing what to expect will lessen the pressure of the ordeal and, more importantly, increase your chances of winning.

Giving a deposition

Knowing what to say, how to act,
and when to remain silent can mean the
difference between bolstering your
credibility and undermining your defense.

"**D**id you review the symptoms of a warfarin overdose with Mr. Rodriguez?" the plaintiff's attorney asked Cindy Fields, RN. Mr. Rodriguez had died of an internal hemorrhage shortly after starting on the anticoagulant. His family claims his death could have been avoided if he'd been told all the warning signs.

"Yes," Fields answered. "I always inform patients about medication side effects and symptoms."

The attorney stared at her and waited. "Besides," Fields continued, "he had already spoken with Dr. Swan, so Mr. Rodriguez would have known the warning signs and the need to call the doctor if they developed."

"How do you know Dr. Swan told him about the warning signs?"

"Because it's her responsibility to give the patient that information."

"So, in other words, you assumed Dr. Swan had told Mr. Rodriguez about the side effects of warfarin—even though the chart had no entry stating that he had been so informed?"

Fields is giving a deposition—an out-of-court recording of sworn testimony by a witness or defendant—and she's made a common mistake: Volunteering information to fill an uncomfortable silence when a simple Yes or No would have sufficed. Now, she's on the defensive, her credibility called into question.

A deposition is a pretrial discovery tool, an opportunity for the attorneys for the plaintiff and the defense to try to find out

as much as possible about the alleged malpractice. It's also a
chance for the lawyers to gauge the strength of each other's case
and how credible a witness you are.

Slipups during a deposition could weaken your position and
come back to haunt you if the case goes to trial, when the
attorney may read parts of your testimony aloud to the judge
and jury. With the stakes high, you need to know what to expect
if you are ever called to give a deposition, and how to put your
best foot forward. (The rules that apply in depositions also apply
in the courtroom if the case goes to trial.)

When you receive notice, mum's the word

As soon as you find out about your involvement in a lawsuit,
notify your hospital attorney or risk manager, as well as your own
malpractice carrier if you have one. If you are named as a
defendant, your personal insurance carrier will probably assign
an attorney to you. In most other instances you'll work with a
lawyer representing your employer.

A claims investigator from your malpractice carrier may be in
frequent contact with you initially. Ask to see identification
before talking to this person.

Do not discuss the case with anyone else unless your lawyer or
insurance representative is present. That includes any co-defendants,
and even fellow nurses on your unit. Although your interests are
ostensibly the same, there is always the potential for conflict.

Under no circumstances call the patient who is suing you or
his attorney. This is a common temptation. Resist it: You could
wind up revealing things the plaintiff wasn't aware of, thereby
strengthening his case against you.

Meet with your attorney as soon as possible, and apprise him
of all facts relating to the case. Do not hold back potentially
damaging information about either the case or about yourself—
a conviction for a crime, for instance, or disciplinary hearings

before the state board. It will hurt you more if the opposing side uncovers and reveals the information before your attorney has had a chance to defuse it.

Your lawyer, in turn, should brief you on who else is involved in the case, what the plaintiff's arguments are likely to be, and, possibly, the approach the opposing attorney is likely to take.

Review the patient's medical record with your lawyer, paying special attention to the care plan, nurses' notes, and any entries you made. If you are not allowed to make copies of relevant documents in the chart, make notes of all pertinent facts.

Look up all relevant policies and procedures in effect at the time of the alleged negligence. Check to see whether your employer's policy manual includes an official statement advising nurses to use independent judgment in carrying out these policies and procedures. You may find a need to refer to this statement at the deposition.

To be certain you are familiar with the standard of care, also carefully review such relevant documents as guidelines from nursing organizations and your state's Nurse Practice Act.

Since a deposition generally takes place months or years after the incident occurred, you may no longer be employed at the same job. If that's the case, review the terminology, abbreviations, and protocols in use at the time.

Because of the lapse of time, you won't be expected to remember every detail of a patient's care, and certain documents will be on hand during the deposition for you to refer to, if necessary. Ask your attorney which ones.

Preparation is your best defense

Some defendants mistakenly think the deposition is their chance to air their entire story—and that once they do the plaintiff will drop the suit. That's highly unlikely, and rattling off unasked for details is almost certain to do more harm than good. You should keep your answers as brief and succinct as possible.

Ideally, much of your testimony should consist of five responses: "Yes," "No," "I don't know," "I don't recall," and "I don't understand the question." Of course, it's not always possible, or wise, to answer this way, but these responses are appropriate more often than you might think.

A practice question-and-answer session with your attorney should be a major part of your preparation. Here are some tips the two of you should cover:

Avoid absolutes. The phrases "I always" and "I never" can box you into a corner if the attorney produces evidence to the contrary. A better response is "It's my customary practice to do it that way."

If necessary, qualify your answer by acknowledging that certain situations may require deviation from normal practice, such as emergencies or instances where the patient's safety is at stake. Be prepared to give specific examples of situations where such deviations may be justified.

Don't guess. Many deponents are afraid of sounding ignorant, so they make a guess when they are unsure of an answer. If you do and are off the mark, you'll come off looking worse than if you had simply been honest and said "I don't remember." If documents are on hand that can refresh your memory, don't be reluctant to ask to see them.

Likewise, if you don't know the answer to a question, say so and stop there. Don't speculate or offer conjecture.

Make sure you use the terms "I don't know" and "I don't remember" correctly: The former means you never knew the information; the latter means that you knew once but have since forgotten.

Don't jump the gun. Many deponents anticipate the next question. As a result, they answer it before it's even asked—and it may never *be* asked. Other deponents volunteer information because they want to be helpful.

You can avoid these mistakes by listening carefully to the question, taking time to analyze it, and answering as narrowly as possible. If you do not understand a question, say so, or ask the attorney to repeat or rephrase it.

Don't be surprised if the opposing attorney stares at you when you finish giving an answer. It's an attempt to get you to say more. Don't; simply sit quietly and wait.

Correct factual errors or wrong assumptions. Your attorney should object to questions containing either of these elements. If he doesn't, ask the plaintiff's attorney to rephrase the question. If it still contains the mistake, correct the misinformation in your answer—not in a remark to the attorney. For example, if you're asked, "On what did you base your diagnosis that the patient had a virus?" An appropriate answer would be "I did not make a diagnosis."

Do not assume that you know what the lawyer meant or his reason for making an incorrect statement; it may simply be that the attorney is unfamiliar with nursing or medicine.

Be wary of hypothetical questions. Your attorney will probably object to these kinds of questions, since they call for speculation. Hypothetical questions are appropriate for expert witnesses, but not for "fact" witnesses.

Since you may have to answer a question despite your attorney's objection, be sure to practice your responses to various hypothetical questions with your attorney beforehand. In many cases, the best answer may simply be, "I don't know."

Body language can speak louder than words

Even though you may feel nervous and intimidated at the deposition, try to at least appear confident. Don't lose your temper. By observing your reactions at the deposition, the plaintiff's lawyer will know exactly which buttons to push at trial.

To help maintain your composure, pause before you speak. Doing so also gives your attorney a chance to object to a question or line of questioning. Listen carefully to the objection;

it may contain a subtle reminder for you. If you need a break to relax, ask for one. (Feel free to ask for a lunch break, too.)

Speak clearly when you answer so the court reporter can hear you. Since your testimony may be read aloud at trial, avoid the use of informal language that may convey a negative image; "Yes" sounds more professional than "Yeah, right."

You should receive a transcript of the proceedings two or three months after you testify. Review it carefully with your attorney and correct any errors you find in it immediately. Remember that the case is still in litigation, so do not discuss it with anyone.

Your thorough preparation for a deposition, straightforward testimony, and prompt follow-up will help ensure a fair legal forum for everyone involved—your former patient, your employer, and you.

Being an expert witness

Interested in testifying as an expert in malpractice cases? Here's what you need to consider before stepping into the witness box.

I t wasn't too long ago that testifying about the appropriateness of a nurse's actions was strictly the domain of doctors. But, as the clinical expertise and autonomy of nurses have grown, so has their legal stature. Today, more and more malpractice attorneys are relying on the words of a nurse to help win their cases.

And it's not just the practices of nurse defendants that RNs now give expert opinions about. In cases where actions are not exclusively within the professional sphere of physicians—the administration of IV meds, for instance—courts have held that nurses are competent to testify as to whether physician defendants met the standard of care.

Given the amount of time nurses spend directly caring for and observing patients, attorneys may even look to an RN to provide expert testimony about a patient's prognosis. That's what a plaintiff's lawyer did in a case a few years ago involving a patient who was taken off life support at an Illinois hospital.

The patient had an advance directive authorizing discontinuation of life support in the event that there was no real hope for recovery. But the patient's family sued the physician who ordered the withdrawal of ventilator support, charging that he had acted too quickly and without due consideration.

At trial, the physician admitted that he had seen the patient for only about 15 minutes a day during the last five days of the patient's life. He also said that he had not consulted with any other physician or nurse regarding the patient's condition and prospects for recovery.

Three of the patient's nurses were called to the stand as experts. Two of them disputed the physician's prognosis, testifying that, based on their experience and professional knowledge, they believed the patient had an even chance of ultimately recovering.

The third nurse wasn't as hopeful about the patient's prognosis, but did testify that, in her opinion, the physician should have waited a few more days before giving the order to disconnect life support.

The testimony of the three nurses may have helped sway the jury, which found for the plaintiff.

Whatever the particulars of a case, the larger legal question that expert witnesses address is always the same: Did the defendant act as a reasonably prudent health care professional with a similar background would have acted under similar circumstances?

Do you suit the case—and does the case suit you?

The only legal requirement you need to testify as a nurse expert is an RN license. But when choosing an expert witness, attorneys look for nurses with additional qualifications, ones that will add weight to their testimony.

The length of time you have been in clinical practice is key. Attorneys generally look for a nurse who has at least five years of current clinical experience, but in some cases, they want 10 years or more.

Your particular field of expertise is equally important. If the alleged malpractice occurred during surgery, for example, an OR nurse rather than, say, an oncology nurse would be called to testify.

Specialty certification, published professional writing, and participation in professional seminars are all relevant. So is your educational level, although often less so than your professional experience.

If a lawyer approaches you about testifying as an expert, he'll provide you with copies of medical records and other relevant documents in the case. Review them carefully. (You'll be paid for the time it takes you.)

After your review, the attorney will ask for your opinion. If it does not support the side he's representing, he won't ask for your services. If it does and he asks you to testify as an expert, don't automatically say Yes. Unlike "fact" witnesses who must testify if subpoenaed, you have no duty to serve as an expert witness.

To decide whether you should or not, ask yourself the following questions:

- Do I firmly agree with the point of view I'm being asked to support? The witness stand is no place to equivocate. If you have any uncertainties about the case you are being asked to help make, decline to testify. That sounds simple but may not be; some lawyers are talented at convincing expert witnesses to see things their way.
- Am I well-versed on the standards of care and authoritative texts in the field? If you're not, you'd be wise not to testify. The opposition lawyer will be looking for knowledge deficits; if he finds any, he'll use them to question your reputation.
- Am I willing and able to devote adequate time to the case? You'll have to figure in pretrial work—including deposition, consultations, and research—preparation for the trial, court appearances, and waiting time. And remember, the case may drag on for months or years.
- Do I feel comfortable with the attorney? If you don't get along with or have confidence in the attorney who is asking you to testify, consider declining the request.
- Will I be compensated fairly? To calculate your hourly fee, multiply the hourly income you receive in your clinical practice by three or four. Request some money up front— perhaps a quarter to a third of what your projected final fee will be. The best way to do this is to write to the lawyer

stating your fee and your requirements concerning advance money and subsequent payment terms. Ask him to endorse the letter and return it to you. This makes a valid, albeit informal, contract.

Avoiding pitfalls when you testify

The first place you'll give testimony is at the deposition. You'll follow the same advice if the case goes to trial. Be frank, of course, but keep your answers brief and succinct; don't volunteer information, and don't stray outside your area of expertise. A practice question-and-answer session with the attorney who asked for your services should be part of your preparation for trial. If the attorney doesn't schedule one, ask for it.

As an expert witness, you will be expected to answer hypothetical questions. To be legally proper, this type of question must contain all relevant facts in evidence in that case—minus names and other precise identifying information—and cannot incorporate things not in evidence.

For example, the lawyer might start by saying: "Assume a 43-year-old patient is hospitalized for (he names a condition) in May, 1993, and that (he continues with the balance of facts in evidence)." You'll then be asked whether the defendant's actions were consistent with the usual and customary practice at the time.

When answering hypothetical questions—as with all others—it's crucial to appear objective and impartial. Avoiding the impression of being a "hired gun," however, can be harder than you think. A nurse in one case, for example, responded to an attorney's hypothetical question by telling him that he had "left out" a certain relevant fact.

Correcting the attorney and revealing that she had knowledge of facts not yet in evidence gave the appearance of bias, and hurt her credibility. The correct response would have been

A personal perspective

As a nurse who's been an expert witness for seven years and consulted on more than 50 cases, I've often found the role rewarding. But I've also encountered difficulties that have soured me on the experience. If you're thinking of serving as an expert witness, here are some things I've learned that you may want to consider:

Be prepared for a lack of consideration, even rudeness, from some judges. Once when I needed to leave court to start my shift in the ED, the judge told me he would hold me in contempt if I left—even though the case had been scheduled to start hours before and I had informed the court ahead of time when I would need to leave and why. I managed to call work to tell them I couldn't come, but the incident was brought up at my next performance evaluation.

Be prepared to have your reputation—and character—attacked by the opposing attorney. In an attempt to diminish your qualifications and uncover a conflict of interest, the questions and insinuations can get personal. I've even been accused of having an affair with the lawyer of one of the parties in a case!

The attorney on whose behalf you are testifying should protect you from such attacks. That's one reason it's so important to be selective about the lawyers you work with. Watch for red flags. For example, does the lawyer return your phone calls in a timely manner? Does he give you the runaround when it comes to payment?

By helping to hold negligent health care professionals accountable, and helping to defend those whose conduct does meet the standard of care, nurses who testify as experts do an important service. But you need to have a thick skin. And you need to go into it with your eyes open.

— **Patricia Carroll,**
RN,C, MS, CEN, RRT

something like "I would need more information to form an opinion. Can you rephrase the question?"

Don't fall into the trap of saying "Yes" if you're asked whether you are being paid for your testimony. Answer that you are being paid for your time and expert knowledge, not for your "testimony."

Pay attention to how you look and act

Your demeanor and appearance are important to establishing your credibility as a witness. Be neat and well-groomed. Wear a conservative suit or dress; do not wear flashy jewelry.

When you are called to come up to the witness stand, stand up straight, face the person administering the oath, and raise your hand with fingers erect. A drooping wrist or halfhearted elevation of the arm looks tentative and unprofessional. Your actions should communicate just the opposite—confidence, forthrightness, and professionalism.

Speak firmly and loudly enough for the court stenographer and jurors to hear you, both when you take the oath and when you begin testifying. Once in the witness chair, keep your feet on the floor; don't cross your legs or fidget. Let your hands rest comfortably in your lap and sit erect with your buttocks well back in the seat. Never slouch.

Being an effective expert witness means combining your nursing knowledge with a measure of legal savvy. Doing that can add another dimension to your professional practice. The courts and the public will benefit from your special knowledge, and you will gain the satisfaction that comes from contributing to the administration of justice.

Q&A:
The Legal Process

About the National Practitioner Data Bank

I was recently named in a negligence suit. Is my name going to show up in the National Practitioner Data Bank, and if so what kind of repercussions can I expect?

If your case is either settled before trial or a jury renders a judgment against you, the party making the payment on your behalf will be required to report that fact to the National Practitioner Data Bank (NPDB). The data bank contains the names of licensed clinical professionals who have had a malpractice payment made on their behalf or who have had an adverse action taken against them professionally.

Besides your name, the NPDB will be given the amount of the payment, the name of the hospital with which you are affiliated, and a description of the act on which the claim is based.

Authorized individuals or entities—such as state licensing boards—may query the data bank and receive a copy of this information. However, hospitals are not required to query the NPDB about a nurse unless she has been granted clinical privileges or belongs to the medical staff, which usually only applies to advanced practice nurses.

It's therefore unlikely that you will suffer any serious repercussions as a result of your name being in the NPDB. It is more likely that you will be asked a question about your involvement in a malpractice action directly—on an employment or insurance application, for example.

Making copies can get you in trouble

I often give copies of helpful clinical articles to fellow nurses— sometimes at inservices, sometimes on a one-to-one basis. Do I need to obtain copyright permission from the publishers of the articles?

Afraid so. Although the "fair use" doctrine allows you to make one copy of an article for personal use, such as your own study or research, making multiple copies for staff constitutes a copyright infringement. Although publishers rarely prosecute violators like you, respecting the publisher's rights is a matter of professional and ethical practice.

If you don't feel like writing to the journal's publisher to request copyright permission, you could always discuss the content of the article with colleagues. Better yet, you could place the journal on reserve in your library so that staff members can read it on their own.

Euthanasia and assisted suicide

I'm confused by the various terms applied to the end-of-life debate. What's the difference between active euthanasia, passive euthanasia, and assisted suicide? And are they all illegal?

Passive euthanasia can be defined as allowing a hopelessly ill or injured person to die, and is usually applied to the withdrawal or withholding of life-sustaining treatment. Active euthanasia is intentionally administering the means of death to another person, such as injecting a patient with a lethal dose of medication. In contrast, assisted suicide is making the means of death available to the patient—like giving him a bottle of barbiturates—while knowing that the patient intends to kill himself.

Since active euthanasia is considered murder, it's obviously against the law. Passive euthanasia, however, is not only legal but health care professionals are duty-bound to comply with patient requests to forego treatment.

As for assisted suicide, most states have specific criminal statutes prohibiting it, and the Supreme Court recently rejected charges that the statutes in New York and Washington were unconstitutional. To date, Oregon is the only state with a law that authorizes physician-assisted suicide, although that law—passed in 1994—still has not been implemented and, in fact, is being sent back for another vote.

Punitive damages: Who must pay?

I read about the size of some punitive damage awards and shake my head because they seem so excessive. When can punitive awards be assessed in cases of nursing malpractice, and do malpractice insurers cover these damages?

Almost all states allow punitive damages in malpractice cases against health care professionals, but the jury must determine that there's been more than ordinary negligence. Many states require a finding of gross negligence; others stipulate that the defendant's conduct must rise to the level of "willful or wanton."

Individual malpractice insurance policies usually do not cover punitive damages. If they did, the defendant would not be punished and others would not be deterred from similar actions.

Depending on the state, punitive damages are sometimes covered in a hospital's or nursing home's policy. The employer may sometimes be assessed for the punitive damages—assuming that the negligence arose out of a duty that was within the nurse's scope of employment. If the nurse was acting outside that scope—she assaulted a patient, for instance—she would be personally responsible for paying any damages.

How safe is your workplace for kids?

Children often accompany their moms to our clinic. Sometimes they're left unattended in the waiting area; sometimes they come into the exam room with their mom. What if the child gets hurt? Who's responsible for supervising them?

The responsibility of supervising children in a clinic or doctor's office is, arguably, the parent's. However, maintaining a "child-safe" office—particularly if it's reasonable to assume that small children will be present—is clearly the responsibility of the clinic or office staff. And that's where liability may lie if a child is injured.

To protect kids from harm and the staff from liability, look at your work environment through a child's eyes. Keep chemical solutions, meds, electrical equipment, sharps, and exam gloves out of the reach of children, or store them in a cabinet with a child-proof lock. If an injury occurs, tell the parent to take the child to a pediatrician, and file an incident report.

Should you speak to a co-defendant's lawyer?

After I was named in a lawsuit filed by a former patient, the attorney for a doctor who was also named called to clarify something I'd written in the patient's chart. Was it wise of me to speak with the lawyer?
Although speaking with the attorney for a co-defendant is usually harmless, it pays to be cautious. There are times when the positions of co-defendants are at odds. If there is a conflict between parties, your lawyer should be present whenever you talk with co-counsel. Since you may not even realize that there's a conflict, always consult with your own attorney before talking with anyone about the substance of the case.

Jury selection: more science than art?

The lawyer my malpractice insurer engaged to defend me in a wrongful death suit wants to use a "jury consultant." If my attorney isn't able to select a jury on his own, maybe I don't have the right lawyer. Should I protest?
Jury consultants—lay people who are experts in evaluating members of the jury pool—are becoming increasingly common in cases where the potential civil or criminal penalties are high. The consultants base their recommendations on a person's body language, facial expressions, general appearance, and other factors believed to reveal a prospective juror's inclinations.

Don't be too concerned by your lawyer's desire to use a jury consultant. If you feel strongly about it, though, discuss the matter with your attorney. If you're still uncomfortable, you can try writing to your insurance company, asking that another attorney be assigned to your case and stating why you object to your present lawyer. Send your letter by certified mail with a return receipt requested.

Be aware, however, that under the provisions of your policy, your insurance company controls your defense; if they deny your request, you'll have to work with the lawyer you have.

Negligence doesn't always mean liability

Can a health care provider be negligent and yet not be liable?
Yes. Only two factors have to be present to establish negligence: a duty owed (the duty to provide care in accordance with prevailing professional standards), and a breach of that duty (a departure from those standards).

To establish liability, though, the plaintiff must prove two additional elements: injury and causation. In other words, the negligent act—or the breach of duty—must have directly caused the injury.

If your employer doesn't report child abuse

I work for a managed care group giving telephone referrals for substance abuse and mental health treatment. If I uncover something during a conversation that leads me to suspect an enrollee is an abusive parent, I note that in the patient record. The medical director then decides whether to file a child abuse report with the state. Often, he decides not to. My employer maintains that RNs who staff the referral line are not mandated to report suspected child abuse because we're not functioning "clinically" and we don't actually see the child. Is that right?
Most, if not all states, require health care professionals to report suspected child abuse. However, specific reporting requirements vary by state. Assuming the statute for your jurisdiction stipulates that a nurse has to gain information "clinically"—and most statutes do not—it sounds like your employer is interpreting the law very narrowly. If you are a professionally licensed nurse taking a health history, you are, in our opinion, functioning clinically.

Company policy can never override statute. Still, it's quite possible that the medical director has a legitimate reason for not reporting certain cases, such as information about the patient you aren't aware of. There are also federal laws that protect the confidentiality of information gained in substance abuse and psychiatric settings. If there isn't a legitimate reason, you have an obligation to report the suspected abuse.

Options in the legal profession

I'm interested in working in the legal profession, but I still want to use my nursing knowledge. What are my options?
You may want to consider becoming a legal nurse consultant. These are RNs who do medical-legal consulting for law firms, government agencies, insurance companies, and risk management departments. Neither a law degree nor paralegal training is required, but nurses must be versed in civil litigation, either through course work in this area or self-study. For information, write to the American Association of Legal Nurse Consultants, 4700 West Lake Ave., Glenview, IL 60025-1485; (847) 375-4713.

If you want to go to law school, you can join the ranks of nurse attorneys—RNs who also have earned their juris doctor, or JD, degree. Many work in areas that use their dual training, such as medical malpractice. To find out more, contact The American Association of Nurse Attorneys, 3525 Ellicott Mills Dr., Suite N, Ellicott City, MD 21043; (410) 418-4800.

Shopping for liability insurance

I'm looking for an insurance policy that will provide coverage for lawsuits filed by patients I cared for in the past. Does this type of insurance exist?
There are two kinds of liability insurance. Occurrence insurance gives you lifetime coverage for anything that occurred during the time you held that policy. Claims-made insurance covers you if the alleged incident occurred after you first purchased the policy and the claim is filed during the time you hold that

policy. If someone sues you after a claims-made policy has expired, you're not covered.

Some insurance companies do allow practitioners to buy retroactive coverage when a claims-made policy is first being written. They generally offer this option only if the practitioner is switching from another carrier's claims-made policy and there is no lapse in his insurance coverage.

That's why it's wise to consider purchasing "tail coverage" when you drop a claims-made policy. This will, in effect, convert the policy to occurrence insurance in terms of covering claims arising from incidents that occurred when you held that policy.

The liability clock stops ticking eventually

A patient threatened to sue when she was injured as a result of a clinical error a year ago, but no legal action was ever taken. How long does she have to file a claim?

The statute of limitations for malpractice varies from state to state. In many, it expires two or three years after the incident, although minors often have at least a year beyond the state's legal age of majority to file suit. Anyone planning to sue the federal government, such as a VA hospital, must do so within two years.

There are a number of exceptions to these limits, though. Patients who had no way of knowing right away about a negligent act that may have resulted in injury, such as surgical patients who have had objects left in them, often get extensions—in some states, a year or more from the time of "discovery." Certain factors that preclude a person from filing suit, such as being in a coma or out of the country, may also extend the statute of limitations.

Declaring death is sometimes a nurse's job

As a home care nurse, can I legally pronounce a patient dead? Often it takes hours before the doctor arrives.

Declaring death used to be strictly the domain of doctors, but in some states nurses can make this pronouncement, too. There are usually stipulations, though. Often, for instance, the nurse can only pronounce in a home care or hospice setting. And in Connecticut, a nurse can declare death only if the patient's doctor previously had written an "anticipated death" order acknowledging that the end of life is imminent.

Your agency should have information about your state law and any restrictions. If the statute permits nurses to declare death, your employer should provide explicit policies for doing so. Be sure to document lack of vital signs and other relevant clinical findings, even when death is expected, and notify the attending physician immediately after the patient dies.

Are Good Samaritan laws always a shield?

While I was visiting at another hospital, an OB nurse who knew I was an RN asked me to assist with an emergency delivery. There was no doctor available and the staff nurses were busy with other patients, so I agreed. Could I have been held liable for negligence if I'd done something wrong?

That depends on your state's Good Samaritan law. While every state has some sort of statute protecting caregivers who render emergency care in good faith, some state laws do not grant immunity for care given in a hospital.

What's more, Good Samaritan laws generally shield you from liability for negligence but not gross negligence. Abandoning the expectant mother after initially coming to her aid might have fallen into that category, since a professional relationship between patient and caregiver was established the moment you started helping.

Because the incident you describe raises serious questions about patient safety at that hospital, you should report it to the facility's administrator or risk manager as well.

Current Controversies

The legal risks of managed care

Just as managed care is still evolving, so are the liability issues it brings. Here's a look at the shape of things to come.

Managed care, in a nutshell, is about managing costs. But by denying or approving payment for health care services, managed care organizations influence much more than the bottom line. Essentially, they, too, participate in patient-care decision making.

That has plenty of nurses worried. They're concerned that the ascendance of managed care will diminish their ability to provide quality care. The public is worried, too, fearing that the desire to control costs will result in delays in diagnosis and denial of treatment.

Such allegations have been the basis of several high-profile lawsuits. HMOs have been slapped with large judgments for refusing to pay for certain treatments, such as bone marrow transplants for cancer patients.

In a recent case that was closely watched by managed care companies, a California jury handed down a $3 million judgment against two HMO-affiliated physicians, finding them negligent in a woman's death from colon cancer.[1] Despite such symptoms as abdominal pain and rectal bleeding, the cancer went undiagnosed for months as the physicians ignored the woman's requests to be referred to a specialist.

The lawyer for the deceased woman's family challenged the HMO's method of paying affiliated physicians, claiming the fact that the two doctors had a financial incentive not to refer patients to specialists played a part in their actions. Although the judge threw out that allegation before jury deliberations began, some courts have held that third-party payers may be liable for the impact of their decisions, such as the denial of payment for hospital care.[2]

Many states are taking a legislative approach to such accountability. In 1995, more than 30 bills regulating managed care companies passed state legislatures.[3]

In New Jersey, for instance, regulations require HMOs to: disclose financial incentives that reward doctors for limiting referrals or hospital admissions, pay for screenings to determine medical emergencies, provide external review of coverage denials, and have continuity of care provisions available when providers are dropped from the network. The regulations also mandate that doctors—not, say, a utilization review coordinator—decide if care should be limited or denied.[4]

While to date most of the liability concerns revolving around managed care have involved physicians and the insurers themselves, nurses are feeling the heat, and have lots of questions. It's still too early to know all of the answers—or even all the issues for that matter—but here is a rundown on what we know so far.

Consider these five hot spots

Some of the legal pitfalls raised by managed care are ones that nurses have traditionally had to sidestep; others represent relatively uncharted waters. Managed care isn't necessarily the sole factor responsible for the issues discussed here, but it's a prime one.

Premature discharge. Under managed care, discharge planning decisions are increasingly being made administratively, not at the bedside. Some nurses fear they are being made arbitrarily, by a cookbook formula, with little regard for the patient's individual needs.

Take, for instance, the one-day hospital stay that had been typically allotted by managed care plans for women after giving birth. Consumer advocates and politicians took aim at that policy, and federal legislation now mandates a two-day stay after normal vaginal delivery and four days after a caesarean, but, for most patients, early discharge is still the rule of the day. Anecdotal reports indicate that, with the managed care organization calling the shots, some hospitals are even sending patients who undergo total hip replacement straight from the recovery room to a nursing home.

As the site of care moves out of the hospital, patients' level of acuity is outstripping the capabilities of nurses in other settings. So, many post-surgical patients who are discharged early wind up right back in the hospital.

To be able to prevent premature discharge in an era of managed care, you must learn who the key decision makers are so you can take your concerns to the right person. That's probably the utilization review coordinator or case manager, working either in the hospital or off-site at the managed care company.

Of course, you would still initially report your concerns to the physician—but that may not be enough. Doctors who sign agreements to participate in networks are under pressure from the managed care plan and the hospital to discharge patients early. You may need to intervene as a patient advocate.

You will need to communicate in succinct, tangible terms the reason a particular patient is not ready to be discharged, and be innovative if your message isn't getting across. One nurse took photographs of a patient and brought them to the utilization review coordinator. The photos put a human face on an abstract condition, and resulted in the patient's continued inpatient treatment.

Downsizing. Not only are patients in the hospital for fewer days, but staff reductions have cut down on the amount of time nurses can spend with each patient—raising concerns about their ability to provide comprehensive, quality care. What's more, layoffs and the increased use of unlicensed assistive personnel mean that more hospital RNs are being asked to supervise non-nurses. That new responsibility brings with it a heightened risk of liability, since RNs can be held accountable for the actions of staff they oversee or to whom they assign work.

To minimize the potential for harm to the patient and liability for yourself, make sure the tasks you delegate are within the UAP's scope of training and in accordance with hospital policy. Also be sure you provide supervision and follow-up as needed. If you are being asked to delegate work you feel is inappropriate or if your workload will prevent you from providing adequate oversight, tell your supervisor—before you begin your shift—that you won't accept the assignment.

Don't forget, there's strength in numbers. At one hospital, all the ICU nurses refused to delegate any professional nursing tasks to a UAP working on the unit, and eventually the hospital removed the UAP from the ICU.[5] Unions representing nurses have also been tackling the UAP issue. Some have won staffing and other quality-of-care guarantees in contracts negotiated with hospitals.

Emergency care. The Emergency Medical Treatment and Active Labor Act (EMTALA), commonly known as the anti-dumping law, requires every hospital that receives federal funds to evaluate and stabilize patients who come to the emergency room. But managed care companies have been refusing to pay for tests ordered for ED patients who, on retrospective review, turn out not to have had a medical emergency.

Hospitals are in a bind. Since they're compelled by federal law to screen patients, nurses and physicians in the ED must continue to do so, even if they aren't reimbursed for it.

There's been consumer and legislative pressure on this front, too, though. A bill introduced in the House of Representatives in 1995 was aimed at requiring all health plans to base payment decisions on the symptoms that bring the patient to the ED, not the ultimate diagnosis. To stave off such action, the American Association of Health Plans, an organization representing the great majority of the nation's managed care plans, announced recently a new policy on emergency care: It states that health plans should cover ED screening and stabilization for conditions that reasonably appear to constitute an emergency, based on the patient's presenting symptoms. It further defines an emergency as a condition that arises suddenly and requires immediate treatment.

Although that seems to resolve the dilemma, managed care companies are not bound to follow the policy. So, unless a hospital is located in a state with a legislative mandate that requires managed care companies to cover ED services, refusals to pay could well continue. And that could lead to cutbacks elsewhere in the facility in an effort to make up for lost revenue.

Licensure. The fact that many managed care organizations operate in more than one state raises a novel question for nurses employed by companies as case managers or utilization review coordinators: Am I functioning purely as an administrator or am I providing professional services?

If the latter, and the nurse is licensed in only one state, conceivably she could be charged in the others with practicing without a license. There is at least one such instance involving a physician—a medical director of a Florida HMO who was licensed in a different state. The physician was charged in Florida with practicing medicine without a license.

A similar issue arises for nurses who staff "dial-a-nurse" telephone lines, which often provide advice to patients in more than one state. Is the nurse just following protocols that appear on a computer screen and therefore not practicing nursing? What if she strays outside protocol, such as when making triage decisions?

Fear alone may force some nurses to stick to a cookbook approach, making the use of independent judgment less likely. However, even this is no sure-fire protection, since the nurse must still use her professional, nursing judgment in determining exactly which "recipe" she should use.

Patient confidentiality. The emergence of managed care networks means that more players than before need information about the patient—hospitals, employers, individual providers, third-party payers, and utilization managers. The growing reliance on electronic transmission of data makes restricting access to confidential health information an even bigger concern.

For your part, any time you receive a request for health information, ask the person making the request to put it in writing on company letterhead. Do not disclose any information without the patient's written authorization. Any such authorization should state specifically who the information will be released to; avoid the use of blanket consent forms.

The times, they are a changing

Until now, professional standards have been the yardstick for determining whether a nurse acted with "reasonable prudence." But, the emphasis on cost-containment is redefining the standard of care. It's quite possible that when a hospital contracts with a managed care company, it may be agreeing to provide a different—even higher—standard of nursing care than those set by the nursing profession.

In a court of law, a nurse will always be judged according to the higher standard. But out in the field, standards seem to conflict and it's not clear which should hold sway—those set by the nursing profession or by the managed care company?

Consider, for example, a nurse who's employed as a case manager by a managed care plan and one who works in the same capacity for a hospital. While the decisions of both reflect the goal of providing quality and cost-effective care, the weight each nurse gives to each of these factors is likely to differ. What is "reasonably prudent" may well depend on which side of the table the nurse is sitting on.

As hospitals continue to downsize and send patients home sooner, it's clear that nurses will take on more responsibility— and with it increased legal risks. That's especially true for those working in discharge planning, case management, and home care. Communication between nurses, physicians, and others in the network will increase to ensure continuity of care.

All this means nurses will need to be courageous enough to articulate their concerns and fulfill their advocacy role, even if that puts them at odds with their employer. They'll have to familiarize themselves with their patients' health plans, including the parameters of coverage and appropriate contact person.

Now more than ever, the patient's health coverage is going to affect his care. Having to factor an insurance plan into the clinical equation is likely to be the most challenging part of clinical decision making.

REFERENCES

1. Ching v. Gaines, Calif Super Ct (Ventura County), No. 137656, 11/15/95.
2. Fiesta, J. (1994). Premature discharge. Nursing Management, 25(4), 17.
3. Page, L. (1995). Market spawns doctor-patient alliances. American Medical News, 38(42), 3.
4. Washburn, L. (1995, November 18). State unveils HMO safeguards. The Record, p. A1.
5. Shindul-Rothschild, J. (1994). Restructuring, redesign, rationing, and nurses' morale: A qualitative study on the impact of competitive financing. Journal of Emergency Nursing, 20(6), 497.

The liability issues of telemedicine

As *"electronic nursing"* becomes more and more prevalent, you need to know how to manage the emerging legal risks.

Interactive TV. Telepathology. E-mail. Teleconsults. A new lingo has entered the vernacular of health care, and it can be summed up in one word: telemedicine.

Also known as telehealth, telemedicine has been heralded as the next wave in health care because of its potential to speed access to care and extend services to underserved, usually rural, areas. The problem, from a legal perspective, is that this horse was out of the gate before officials sounded the starting gun.

At least 416 rural hospitals already have telemedicine programs up and running, and another 564 facilities have plans to establish a program in the next few years. Federal regulators, legislators, and health care providers have been struggling to keep up with telemedicine's advances, considering ways to remove legal obstacles for clinicians and safeguard the rights of patients.

With the electronic revolution changing the way care is delivered, you'll want to know how telemedicine is being used and what legal signposts dot the road so far.

What exactly is telemedicine?

Telemedicine is the use of communications technology to transmit health information from one location to another. It includes the transmission of radiographic and pathologic images (teleradiology and telepathology) and—more familiar to nurses—telemetry and telephone triage.

One of the most promising applications of telemedicine involves two-way video. At the Medical College of Georgia Telemedicine Center, for example, both the health care provider and the patient sit in front of a camera mounted on top of a desktop computer at their respective locations—often miles apart. They can see, hear, and talk to one another in real time. Interactive TV works the same way, except it utilizes two-way cable television.

Even diagnostic equipment such as a stethoscope or otoscope—referred to as peripherals—can be included in a telemedicine hook-up, enabling the transmission of accompanying sounds and visual images.

A home health nurse at a distant site, for example, can use telemedicine to watch her patient take his blood pressure, change a wound dressing, or administer his own IV therapy. Alternatively, she can be at the patient's side during the video consult, performing a hands-on assessment or wielding peripherals while images are transmitted to a physician specialist at another location.

In yet another application of telemedicine, an ED nurse can monitor via video what's happening to a patient being transported in an ambulance equipped with cameras.

Providing care across state lines

With telemedicine, a provider can just as easily care for a patient who lives across the country as one who lives across town. That ability has led to a key legal question: If I'm licensed to practice in one state and I provide services via telemedicine to a patient in another state, am I breaking the law?

This is hardly an abstract concern. Nurses who staff telephone advice lines for multistate hospital networks or managed care plans with enrollees nationwide regularly provide health information to patients in states where they are not licensed to practice.

As yet, no laws exist that specifically address licensure

requirements for RNs providing services across state lines. Your safest course of action, then, is to obtain licenses in the states where your patients reside. Of course that may not be practical—with some managed care plans, patients may be calling from virtually anywhere.

It would probably be wise, then, to consult with the licensing boards in your own and your patients' states before providing care across state lines. Also check your employer's policy on nursing licensure, or ask your employer's legal counsel about this issue. Try to obtain a copy of the policy or an opinion in writing, whenever possible. Following the advice and having it on paper could help you ward off disciplinary action—or a lawsuit—down the road.

There's yet a secondary issue nurses need to consider: Should a nurse licensed in the patient's state implement orders from an out-of-state physician—one who's not licensed in the state where the patient resides?

Before you follow orders from an out-of-state physician, check your state laws and review any opinions from your state attorney general's office. In one opinion letter, for example, the Mississippi Attorney General decided that physicians located in another state must also be licensed in Mississippi if they give orders that will be administered by a nurse in the state. Although there was no explicit reference made to the liability of a nurse following such orders, it implied that a nurse may not be obligated to follow orders from an out-of-state physician not licensed in Mississippi.

You should also check to see if your state nursing board has issued a ruling on implementing orders from physicians not licensed in the state. If so, following this ruling will allow you to avoid disciplinary action. If the board has been silent on this issue, check your employer's policy or consult with its legal counsel.

In the future, nurses and other providers may get the concrete guidance they need. The National Council of State Boards of Nursing is currently exploring the idea of multistate licensure, which would give nurses the legal authority to practice in participating states without the hassle of obtaining licenses by endorsement.

Efforts like this are being watched closely on the federal level. Under the auspices of the Department of Health and Human Services, the Joint Working Group on Telemedicine—a group charged with developing national policies on telemedicine and reporting its findings to Vice President Al Gore and to Congress—is looking for ways to reduce cross-state licensure burdens for providers.

Meanwhile, the Senate is currently considering a measure that would eliminate another stumbling block to telemedicine: The Medicare requirement that care be provided face-to-face in order to be reimbursable.

A new procedure, a patient's consent

No matter how good telemedicine is, it can't duplicate in-person contact. For that reason, it's a good idea to make sure the patient understands the risks and benefits of the technology so he can make an informed decision about whether to use it.

When using two-way video, for instance, explain that the physician's diagnosis will be based on a transmitted image that may not be as clear as the human eye. And, the telemedicine provider may not have access to senses such as touch and smell. On the other hand, the patient won't have to travel a long distance to receive care.

In 1996, California became the first state to require providers to obtain informed consent—both verbal and written—before delivering non-emergency care via telemedicine. Arizona has signed into law similar legislation and, at press time, Oklahoma is considering it.

As part of California's informed consent requirement, the provider in charge of the patient's care must inform the patient of the risks and benefits of telemedicine both verbally and in writing. The patient must also be informed, among other things, that he will have reasonable access to all information that's transmitted and that it will be protected by existing confidentiality rules.

Failure to meet these requirements could lead to charges of unprofessional conduct. Check your state law or with your employer to see what informed consent requirements must be fulfilled before providing care to a patient using telemedicine. As in providing any care, you should be sure the patient understands the plan of care and that his consent has been documented in his chart.

For your own protection, document your activities and assessment findings whenever you assist a physician during a telemedicine procedure. This is especially important if the consulting physician will be relying on your senses—smell or touch—to help make a diagnosis.

Whether you are at the patient's side or monitoring him from another site, chart what you see, what he tells you, and any instructions you provide. Store all medical data transmissions, like telemetry printouts or videotapes, in the patient's chart.

When assessing and evaluating patients over the phone, you can minimize your risks by following specific protocols or standing orders.

Confidentiality in an electronic age

Most telemedicine laws, either pending or enacted, require providers to uphold existing confidentiality requirements. But they do not specify how to protect the security of electronic transmissions. So, nurses and other providers need to use common sense to protect their patients' privacy.

If your hospital has a telemedicine program, in all likelihood it has already taken steps to ensure the security of electronic data as it's transmitted. Check with the head of the program or your risk manager to see if video, audio, and data transmissions go over fiber optic lines—as opposed to the copper wires used to transmit telephone calls. Fiber optic lines are much more difficult to "tap."

Avoid using e-mail to transmit or receive patient data over the Internet unless your computer is programmed to send and receive messages "in code" using encryption technology. If appropriate, verify the authenticity of messages before responding.

When participating in two-way video consults, inform the patient if anyone is observing the interaction—other providers who are off-camera, for example. Try to ensure that only those who need to know about the patient's condition are present.

Your facility should have a policy for storing information gathered using this technology. To be on the safe side, keep video- and audiotapes and backup computer disks in a secure place for the same amount of time you would store paper records.

Finally, all staff should receive regular updates and refresher courses on avoiding confidentiality breaches in an evolving electronic environment.

The legal concerns presented by telemedicine will continue to unfold. Staying abreast of the issues is the first and most important step in managing your risks.

References

1. Office of Rural Health Policy, U.S. Department of Health and Human Services. (1997, February). Exploratory evaluation of rural applications of telemedicine. Rockville, MD: Author.
2. Telemedicine Research Center. (1997). What is telemedicine? Portland, OR:

HIV and the law: An update

Here's a look at recent legal developments that will affect the way you and other providers care for patients with HIV.

B etween 1991 and 1996, at least 300 legal battles in which HIV or AIDS was a central issue were litigated in the courts.[1] In the legislative arena, an increasing number of statutes dealing with HIV and AIDS have been enacted by lawmakers.

Among the specific issues that courts and legislators have been grappling with: the confidentiality of a person's HIV-related information versus the need for disclosure, mandatory versus voluntary HIV testing, and a patient's right to receive care versus a provider's right to deny it.

Who has the right to know?

If a patient is seropositive or has AIDS, does his status have to be reported to the health authorities? To his caregivers? How about to his spouse?

All 50 states require reporting of AIDS cases—without the patient's consent—to the Centers for Disease Control and Prevention or the state health department for epidemiological purposes. Some states require the reporting of specific data such as the patient's name, address, sex, or age. Others prohibit the disclosure of any identifying information.[2]

To date, there are 26 states* that also require the reporting—by name—of all people diagnosed with HIV. Two others—

*Alabama, Arizona, Arkansas, Colorado, Idaho, Indiana, Louisiana, Michigan, Minnesota, Mississippi, Missouri, Nebraska, Nevada, New Jersey, North Carolina, North Dakota, Ohio, Oklahoma, South Carolina, South Dakota, Tennessee, Utah, Virginia, West Virginia, Wisconsin, Wyoming.

Connecticut, and Texas—require the reporting of HIV infection only in children who are less than 13 years of age.[3] Oregon became the latest state to enact reporting requirements for HIV infection in children; in that state, it applies to children under the age of 6.

Beyond the CDC or state authority, however, state confidentiality statutes generally prohibit the disclosure of HIV-related information to anyone who is not a health care provider without the patient's consent, and courts have upheld these statutes.

In Washington, D.C., for example, one court's controversial ruling held that the staff of a mental health facility had no duty to inform the husband of a patient that his wife had tested positive for HIV. Their duty was solely to the patient—and they were to refrain from disclosing the woman's test results to anyone without her written consent or by order of the court.[4]

In the last several years, however, an increasing number of legislatures and courts have carved out exceptions to strict confidentiality rules, permitting disclosure of HIV-related information to those who have a "need to know."

Who falls into this category varies by state, and some statutes are more specific than others. Most states do, however, allow disclosure to medical personnel who are involved in the patient's treatment. But that does not necessarily mean all of a patient's caregivers. Some states, like California, permit disclosure to anyone who provides direct care to the patient. Others, like Kentucky, limit disclosure to the patient's treating or personal physician.[2]

There are some states that have taken a much less restrictive approach, extending the right to know to those who are deemed at risk for HIV infection. Depending on the state, this may include not only the patient's caregivers but also emergency medical personnel, morticians, and the patient's spouse.

Note, however, that while many of these statutes permit disclosure of a patient's status in certain instances, they do not mandate it. The decision on whether to reveal this information and to whom is usually outlined in local statutes and in the policies and procedures manual of each facility. But, generally, the responsibility is left up to the physician or local health officer.

Taking steps to prevent improper disclosure

While the laws on who should be privy to a patient's HIV/AIDS status are murky at times, one thing is crystal clear: Anyone who reveals information about a patient's HIV status could face both civil liability and disciplinary action for unauthorized disclosure of confidential information.

Do not discuss your patient's health status with anyone other than the patient, his physician, or other direct caregivers unless the patient has given you explicit permission. Check with your facility's risk manager or your supervisor to find out who is authorized to inform those with a need to know.

Whenever a patient's consent is needed to disclose health information, make sure it is in writing. It must specifically indicate what information will be released, to whom, and for how long the consent is valid. (When you are releasing HIV-related data, make sure that it's accompanied by a statement that prohibits the receiving party from further disclosing the information without the patient's explicit consent.)

As with any patient, don't discuss his health in a public area where others may overhear you. If you're giving HIV-related instructions to the patient, for example, take him to a private room.

Your facility may have a confidential means of documenting HIV-related information—say, using a certain code or sticker in the patient's chart. You'll still need to be discreet, though. Don't, for example, place a red sticker with "HIV" or "AIDS" written on the front of the patient's chart and then hang it on the door or leave it in the patient's room.

Remember, too, that you have a duty to advocate for the patient. That means you should report any incidents where you suspect that your patient's health information has been disclosed improperly or without authorization.

Mandatory testing: Where are we headed?

Compulsory HIV testing is generally prohibited, except among certain groups such as military personnel and federal prisoners.[5] Some states, however, do allow HIV testing of patients—without their consent—in cases of accidental exposure.

Still, most professional health organizations—including the ANA and the American Hospital Association—as well as the CDC and the Public Health Service do not support mandatory testing under any circumstances. They argue that it would violate patients' privacy and autonomy, undermine trust in the patient-provider relationship, and dissuade people who may be infected from seeking care.

But in July of 1996, the American Medical Association broke ranks and endorsed mandatory testing of pregnant women and newborns. And, in February of 1997, New York became the first state in the nation to mandate the screening of all newborns for HIV and the disclosure of test results to their mothers.

New York had been testing newborns anonymously for epidemiological purposes. Proponents of the new law argued that it made no sense to discharge babies who tested positive without informing the mother.[5]

Supporters of such legislation argue that early identification and treatment of HIV saves lives. Administering zidovudine (formerly known as AZT) prenatally and to the newborn has recently been shown to significantly reduce the incidence of perinatal transmission.[6]

Other states are likely to follow New York's lead—especially in light of additional financial incentives. Under federal legislation that was passed in 1996, funds from the Ryan White Care Act will be withheld from states that do not do one of the following by March 2000: reduce the number of perinatally transmitted

AIDS cases by 50% compared to 1993 levels, test 95% of women
who receive prenatal care, or mandate testing of all newborns
whose mothers did not undergo prenatal HIV testing.

Personal safety vs. your duty to care

The Americans with Disabilities Act prohibits "public accommodations"—including hospitals and clinics—from discriminating
against people with infectious diseases in their access to services.
The Rehabilitation Act imposes the same duty on health care
facilities that receive Medicare and other federal funds.

Some attorneys argue that small medical offices that operate
on an appointment basis may not be considered places of public
accommodation under federal and state statutes. If that's the
case, they can treat—or not treat—whomever they like. Private
duty nurses can do the same.[7]

Nurses who work for walk-in clinics, home health agencies, or
hospitals, on the other hand—like their employers—generally
lack the legal backing to deny care to a patient with HIV/AIDS.
Refusing to care for a patient could result in a charge of insub-
ordination or outright dismissal.

Take the case of a pregnant home health nurse in Alabama
who refused to care for an HIV-positive patient. She felt that her
fetus was vulnerable to infection because she was in her first
trimester and had gestational diabetes, which can weaken the
immune system. The agency had a policy that said that refusal to
treat a patient was grounds for dismissal and the nurse was fired.[7]

The nurse sued her employer, claiming that she'd been
discriminated against because she was pregnant. But a court
ruled for the employer, finding that it had treated pregnant and
nonpregnant staffers who refused to care for HIV-infected
patients alike.

The bottom line: You can ask for a different assignment if you
do not want to care for a patient with HIV—just as you can in
any other situation—but your employer isn't obligated to honor

your request. If, however, your employer has a policy that allows staffers to be reassigned in certain circumstances—say, it permits immunosuppressed nurses to decline assignments to infected patients—then that policy must be applied fairly and consistently.

There are few clear answers to the issues raised by HIV and AIDS—and public policy in this area continues to evolve. Staying current with the laws and court rulings in your state, as well as your own employer's policies, will help you keep out of legal trouble.

REFERENCES

1. Gostin, L. O. (1996, July) The AIDS Litigation Project III: A Look at HIV/AIDS in the Courts of the 1990s. Washington, DC: Kaiser Family Foundation.
2. Brooke, P. (1995). Legal issues related to the care of persons with HIV. In J. H. Flaskerud & P. J. Ungvarski (Eds.), HIV/AIDS: A guide to nursing care (pp. 389-404). Philadelphia: W. B. Saunders.
3. Centers for Disease Control and Prevention. (1996). HIV/AIDS Surveillance Report, 8(1), 3.
4. N.O.L. v. District of Columbia, 674 a.2d 498, (D.C. App. 1995).
5. Staff. (1996, November). Is it time . . . American Medical News, 39(33), 13.
6. Centers for Disease Control and Prevention. (1994). Recommendations of the U.S. Public Health Service Task Force on the use of zidovudine to reduce perinatal transmission of human immunodeficiency virus. MMWR, 43(RR-11), 1.
7. Fowler, M. D., & Chaney, E. A. (1989). Ethical and legal issues. In J. H. Flaskerud (Ed.), AIDS/HIV Infection: A reference guide for nursing professionals (pp. 215-229). Philadelphia: W. B. Saunders.
8. Armstrong v. Flowers Hospital, 33 F.3d 1308, (U.S. App. 1993).

DNR orders: your rights and responsibilities

This "case study" illustrates what can happen when prevailing medical standards and the absence of a DNR order collide with a nurse's advocacy role.

T he standard of care requires nurses to attempt to resuscitate any patient who does not have a Do Not Resuscitate (DNR) order. But what should a nurse do if she believes that resuscitation is inappropriate for her patient?

The safe, easy answer is to resuscitate first and ask questions later; life-sustaining treatments can always be withdrawn. The problem with this solution is that it ignores the nurse's role as patient advocate.

That's a role one nurse thought she was fulfilling when she decided not to begin CPR on a patient under her care. Her decision taught her some tough lessons that all nurses can benefit from hearing.

A clear clinical case, unexpected results

Pat, an RN with 10 years of clinical experience, worked nights at a small community hospital in Virginia. (Certain identifiable facts in this case have been changed to protect the anonymity of both the nurse and the patient.) Mrs. Wilson, a frail, elderly nursing home resident, was well known to Pat and the rest of the hospital staff. She was ventilator-dependent and had multiple medical problems, including hypertension, chronic obstructive pulmonary disease, and a degenerative muscular disease.

On this particular day, Mrs. Wilson had been admitted for insertion of a new endotracheal tube. Several years before, her doctor had asked her if she would want to be resuscitated if she arrested. Mrs. Wilson had refused to discuss the subject. She had no advance directive and had not appointed a surrogate decision-maker.

Following the tube change, Mrs. Wilson's blood pressure dropped. Her pressure was stabilized but the doctor decided to keep her in the hospital overnight for observation.

Shortly after report that evening, Pat entered Mrs. Wilson's room and found that she was extubated. She had no spontaneous respirations, no pulse, and no blood pressure. Her skin was cold and mottled. Her pupils were fixed and dilated.

Pat knew that Mrs. Wilson did not have a DNR order. She also knew that she was dead. So instead of doing CPR, and knowing there were no doctors in-house at the time, Pat telephoned Mrs. Wilson's attending physician. She advised him of Mrs. Wilson's condition, and he agreed that resuscitation would be pointless.

Pat told the other nursing staff not to start resuscitation and directed them to begin post-mortem care. When the patient's family arrived, Pat described what had happened and provided comfort and support.

The following day Pat was called to her supervisor's office and fired. The nursing assistants who followed Pat's instructions not to begin resuscitation were suspended for three days.

Pat's supervisor told her that the hospital's insurer would not defend her if a lawsuit arose, because she had willfully disregarded hospital policy. The Director of Nursing notified the local prosecutor's office of Pat's actions so they could investigate a possible manslaughter charge. The DON also reported Pat to the state board of nursing for possible disciplinary action.

Why the huge fallout? In Virginia—as in most, if not all states—only a physician is allowed to pronounce the death of a hospital patient. As far as the law was concerned, Mrs. Wilson wasn't dead when Pat discovered her, because no physician had pronounced her to be.

Resuscitation decisions and the law

State statutes addressing the withholding and withdrawal of medical care are relatively new; many have been enacted only as recently as the late 1980s. According to *Choice in Dying*, about 27 states have enacted laws dealing with nonhospital DNR orders; these laws typically allow EMS personnel to withhold CPR in certain situations.

But many advance directive statutes either don't mention or only briefly discuss the far more common DNR order used in hospitals or nursing homes. Such laws do little to address the difficult questions nurses and doctors face, especially in light of the statistical futility of resuscitating certain patients: Under what circumstances must resuscitation be done? And when may someone other than the patient decide to withhold resuscitation?

New York, Georgia, and West Virginia are among the minority of states that do address these questions. They also give statutory teeth to what has become common practice: The law in these states says that a person is presumed to have consented to resuscitation in the absence of a DNR order.

New York's law—one of the most comprehensive DNR statutes in the country—details the decision-making authority of patients, surrogates, and attending physicians, taking into account a variety of circumstances. If, for example, an attending physician

After the dust settles, mixed results

Pat appealed to her employer in an effort to regain her job, arguing that she had not violated the hospital's DNR policy. That policy stated that the decision not to resuscitate must be authorized by a physician, be medically, legally, and ethically appropriate, and should be considered when resuscitation is not expected to alter the ultimate outcome and would serve only to prolong the moment of death.

Pat contended that by immediately calling the doctor—who agreed that resuscitation was not warranted—these policy conditions had been met. Be that as it may, the hospital was concerned about appearances—namely, the appearance that a determines that discussing CPR with the patient would cause her severe injury, he may issue a DNR order without the patient's consent, after complying with certain conditions.[1]

When hospitals haven't found the answers they were looking for in their state's law, some have petitioned the courts. One noteworthy case—that of Baby K—involved an infant born with anencephaly who required repeated trips to the hospital for life-sustaining ventilator treatment.[2] When the mother would not consent to a DNR order, the hospital sought a court order to permit it to withhold ventilator treatment the next time the baby returned to the ED in respiratory distress.

A U.S. district court held that the hospital could not withhold treatment—even if such treatment were futile or inhumane—because the Emergency Medical Treatment and Active Labor Act (EMTALA) does not make any exceptions to its requirement to stabilize patients.

Although the ruling was narrow, it reflects a general reluctance on the part of the courts to override the wishes of family members seeking to keep terminally ill or irreversibly unconscious loved ones alive—provided there's no evidence that the patient would have wanted otherwise.

REFERENCE
1. Public Health Law, Article 29-B, Orders Not to Resuscitate. NY CLS Pub Health @ 2960-2979.
2. In the Matter of Baby K. 832 F. Supp. 1022; 1993 U.S. Dist.

nurse had the authority to decide whether a patient should be resuscitated. The supervisor noted that Pat was an "at will" employee, who could be fired for a good reason, a bad reason, or no reason.

Pat would remain an ex-employee

Despite the supervisor's statement that the hospital would not defend Pat in a lawsuit, the hospital was legally liable for Pat's actions, since she had been acting within the scope of her employment. Mrs. Wilson's family did file a lawsuit but, ironically, not against Pat for her failure to resuscitate. Instead, they sued the hospital, the physician, and several other nurses, alleging that the ET tube had been inserted improperly and that the nurses' failure to monitor Mrs. Wilson post-insertion had resulted in her self-extubation.

After the police spoke to Pat and the attending physician—who supported Pat's assertion that Mrs. Wilson was dead when she entered the room—no criminal charges were filed. But professionally, Pat wasn't off the hook. More than a year after the incident, Pat was called before the Board of Nursing. She was accused of negligence, unprofessional and unethical conduct, and posing a danger to the health and safety of a patient.

The letter of the law

In her hearing before the board, Pat argued that the doctor's ratification of her assessment that Mrs. Wilson was dead relieved her of any duty to resuscitate. Although Pat hadn't known it when Mrs. Wilson died, the language in Virginia's statute on the determination of death was on her side: It states that death occurs when a physician determines there is an irreversible cessation of vital functions. It does not require that the physician make that determination first-hand.

There is no legal—and Pat asserted no ethical—duty to resuscitate a dead person. So, Pat argued, she had been neither unprofessional nor negligent. And she hadn't endangered her patient, because Mrs. Wilson was already dead.

One board member did reproach Pat for "failing to act as a patient advocate." ANA's position statement on DNR decisions imposes a duty on nurses to educate the patient and family about treatment decisions.[1] Pat conceded that she and the other members of the health care team should have made a greater effort to learn Mrs. Wilson's wishes over the years, especially as her condition deteriorated.

According to the prevailing standard of care, if a patient's wishes aren't known or ascertainable, treatment decisions must be guided by the patient's best interests. When Pat discovered

Mrs. Wilson's body, she believed that a dignified death—without the severe trauma to Mrs. Wilson's frail body that CPR would have caused—was in her patient's best interests. And, Pat maintained, she had acted in accord with those interests.

The board agreed. Pat was exonerated of all charges.

A proactive approach to avoiding problems

Pat was fortunate that her actions didn't violate Virginia statute. Otherwise, the outcome would have been different. Her case highlights how important it is that nurses know their particular state's laws and their patients' wishes.

You need to ascertain those wishes before an emergency arises, and not rely on doctors to do it—many are reluctant to raise the sensitive subject of DNR orders and advance directives. Explain to patients and families what a DNR order is, and encourage those who request such an order to ask the physician whether the order has, in fact, been written.

Even if a patient does not want any formal advance directive written, nurses and doctors can document patient statements regarding life-sustaining measures in the progress notes. These notes can assist you in knowing what position to advocate for.

If the patient can no longer communicate and there is no surrogate decision-maker, try to determine what types of treatments the patient would want by talking to relatives or friends. Be aware, however, that family members often disagree and may be personally opposed to the withholding of treatment despite the patient's wishes.

Nurses have a duty to honor advance directives, and many statutes provide immunity to health care providers who do. Failing to honor an advance directive—resuscitating a patient who has a DNR order, for example—could lead to a battery suit by the patient or his family, and disciplinary action by the Board of Nursing.

Do your best to ensure that caregivers are aware of any DNR orders that have been written. Flag the patient's chart and the Kardex. Consider "flagging" the patient, such as by using a wrist band of a specially designated color.

Besides knowing your patient's wishes, familiarize yourself with your state's laws on advance directives, resuscitation decisions, and the determination of death. Can a nurse honor an advance directive to withhold resuscitation in the absence of a doctor's order? Can a nurse declare patients dead and, if so, under what circumstances?

With more patients being treated at home and fewer physicians making house calls, a number of states now allow nurses to pronounce death in nonhospital settings—home, hospice, or nursing home. Generally, the nurse can do so only if the patient's doctor has written an "anticipated death" order acknowledging that the end of life is imminent. Other restrictions may need to be met as well.

Even when a death is expected, notify the attending physician immediately after the patient dies, and document the absence of vital signs and other relevant clinical findings.

Finally, read your employer's DNR policy—the JCAHO requires hospitals to have one. Read the ANA position statement on do not resuscitate decisions. Read up on relevant cases that have been decided in your state. Do these decisions and policies promote or impede the role of the nurse as patient advocate?

Statutes, institutional policies, case law, and the codes or position papers of professional associations define your duty. You owe it to yourself and your patients to keep abreast of this material, and to keep the lines of communication between the patient, family, and health care team open at all times.

REFERENCES

1. American Nurses Association. (1992). Position statement on nursing care and do not resuscitate decisions. Washington, DC: Author.

Assisted suicide: Should the patient decide when to die?

With the movement to legalize assisted suicide growing, nurses need to be well-versed in this controversial issue—and their role in caring for terminally ill patients.

I n November of 1994, Oregon voters passed an initiative legalizing physician-assisted suicide. It was an historic moment: Enactment of the Death with Dignity Act would have made Oregon the only place in the world where it is legal to help a person end his life. (Euthanasia is still technically illegal in the Netherlands, although physicians who follow certain guidelines are not prosecuted.) But the law was never enacted. It's been tied up with court challenges and, most recently, has been put back on the ballot for another vote.

The Oregon referendum was relegated to "old news," however, when, in the fall of 1996, the U.S. Supreme Court agreed to hear appeals on two cases that examined whether there's a constitutional right to assisted suicide.

The cases challenged state laws banning assisted suicide in Washington and New York. In the Washington case, the 9th Circuit Court had struck down the law, ruling that "a liberty interest exists in the choice of how and when one dies, and that the provision of the Washington statute banning assisted suicide, as applied to competent, terminally ill adults who wish to hasten their deaths by obtaining medication prescribed by their doctors, violates the Due Process clause (of the U.S. Constitution)."[1]

In the New York case, the 2nd Circuit Court used the equal protection clause of the Constitution to overturn that state's law,

Sorting out the terminology

Assisted suicide is knowingly providing a person with the means to take his own life, such as giving him a prescription for a lethal dose of medicine. The medication or other means of death is self-administered.

Active euthanasia is actually administering the means of death to another person, with the
intention of ending that person's life. For example, injecting a patient with potassium chloride to induce ventricular fibrillation.

Passive euthanasia is a term often applied to withholding or withdrawing a life-sustaining treatment. However, many people find the term inappropriate and confusing. Withdrawing or
withholding an intervention may indeed hasten or cause death; but the intention is to allow the natural process of dying to occur.

There's another big difference: There is legal support for complying with patients' requests to forego interventions. The Supreme Court's landmark Cruzan decision (Cruzan v. Director, Missouri Department of Health, 110 S. Ct. 2841 [1990].) upheld the principle that competent patients have the right to refuse life-sustaining treatments, including artificial nutrition and hydration.[1]

arguing that since those on life support can terminate their treatment, effectively choosing death, it was unconstitutional to deny that right to the terminally ill who aren't on life support. Said the court, "We [hold] that physicians who are willing to do so may prescribe drugs to be self-administered by mentally competent patients who seek to end lives during the final stages of a terminal illness."[2]

The Supreme Court decision, delivered in June, reversed the lower courts, ruling unanimously, that the state laws were not unconstitutional on the grounds presented.

That decision, though historic, is unlikely to settle the question. Experts predict—and the official opinion, written by Chief Justice William Rehnquist, and concurring opinions of other justices seem to indicate—that the debate should and will be continued in state courts and legislatures on grounds other than the narrow ones brought by these two cases.

In fact, about a dozen states have drafted or introduced bills similar to the Oregon initiative. In other states, though, lawmakers have been considering measures to strengthen bans on assisted suicide. And two bills were introduced in Congress in the fall of 1996 to prohibit use of federal funds in assisted suicide.

As the debate goes on, nurses—and the associations that represent them—are finding themselves confronted with one of the most difficult issues of our time.

Death with dignity: model legislation

Before the first Oregon initiative—which passed by a vote of 51% to 49%—measures to legalize physician-assisted suicide had come to ballot in two other states: Washington in 1991 and California one year later. Both measures were narrowly defeated.

Oregon's Death with Dignity Act, the only one with concrete shape, serves, at least, as a blueprint for a law voters would accept, at least once. It would permit a physician to write a lethal drug prescription for a competent, terminally ill adult who is a resident of the state. Other provisions were mandated as well:

- Both the attending and a consulting physician must certify that the patient has no more than six months to live.
- The patient must make both an oral and a written request for the prescription. Those must be followed by a second oral request 15 days or more after the first.
- The attending physician must refer the patient for counseling if a psychological illness or depression is suspected.
- The doctor must wait at least 48 hours after the third request before providing the lethal prescription.

The act grants immunity from civil and criminal liability and protection against professional sanctions to any health care provider—and that would include nurses—who follows the provisions of the law in good faith. The same immunity is extended to those who refuse to participate in a patient's request for assisted suicide. Acts of negligence or willful misconduct are not shielded.

Assisted-suicide laws proposed in other states resemble Oregon's initiative. But some of them, including those defeated in Washington and California, have gone further: They would permit doctors not only to write lethal prescriptions but, in some cases, to administer lethal injections.

The arguments and nursing's stand

Most criminal laws are founded on the belief that the state has a duty to protect life. But right-to-die advocates maintain that there are circumstances in which life is worse than death. They argue that society has a responsibility to relieve unendurable pain and suffering if that's what an individual wants, basing their position on the principles of compassion and beneficence—the duty to do good.

Proponents of assisted suicide also maintain that patients' recognized right to autonomy includes the right to determine how and when they will die. Indeed, part of the groundswell of support for assisted suicide can be ascribed to the public's perception of having little control over end-of-life treatment decisions. That's a concern the Patient Self-Determination Act was supposed to assuage, but it's largely failed to do so.[3]

Opponents argue that if assisted suicide is legalized, less attention will be paid to palliative care, such as more aggressive and effective pain management—a goal the Supreme Court justices advocated in their decision on the Washington and New York cases. They worry about groups such as the elderly and the uninsured, who may be coerced into asking to be killed. Because of this potential for abuse, opponents argue, voluntary assisted suicide is the first step down the "slippery slope" toward involuntary euthanasia.

They cite the principle of nonmaleficence, too, which obligates health care providers to inflict no harm while implicitly promising to protect patients from unnecessary suffering or death.

The ANA officially opposes nurses' participation in assisted suicide and active euthanasia[4,5] because it violates the ethical traditions embodied in the *Code for Nurses*, which states that "the nurse does not act deliberately to terminate the life of any person."[6]

Despite the national association's official position, state groups have not always fallen into line. The California Nurses Association actively opposed the state's 1992 death with dignity referendum, but the nurses' associations in Oregon and Washington state took no official stand when the measures came to ballot in their states.

The nurses' association in Michigan, where Dr. Jack Kevorkian has participated in some two dozen suicides, has come out in support of the legalization of assisted suicide. MNA favors legalization for "competent persons whose suffering cannot be relieved or satisfactorily reduced with alternative strategies."[7]

One on one, what should you do?

If a patient asks you—either directly or indirectly—to help him commit suicide, you are legally obligated to refuse. But there may be a great deal you can do for him, so look for factors that could be affecting his state of mind, such as depression or medication-induced delirium.

Never accept such a request at its face value. He may really be expressing a need for greater control over his pain or his environment. Or his request may be a desperate cry for attention, prompted by fears of a terrible death.

Talk with the patient to find out more. Make sure that your statements and tone are nonthreatening and nonjudgmental. Ask him why he wants to end his life. Validate his concerns about pain or treatments, and try to correct any misconceptions.

Be clear about his options, though. Let him know that the law prohibits you from doing what he is asking but that he always has the right to refuse burdensome or unwanted treatments. Ask if he has filled out an advance directive; if he hasn't but would like to, follow your hospital's procedures for getting this done.

If he is suffering from pain, discuss more aggressive pain control and other ways to manage symptoms more effectively. Communicate his needs and concerns to the physician and your supervisor.

Some patients may want to die because they worry about being too much of a burden on their loved ones. If that's the case, ask the patient if he would like you to arrange for a chaplain or social worker to talk to the entire family.

After your discussion, tell the patient that you need to chart his request to help end his life; explain that this allows his nurses and doctors to better meet his needs. If he objects, evaluate how pertinent the information is to the patient's care and then decide whether or not to honor his wishes. If you decide that you can't, let the patient know.

Ethically and legally, charting what a patient has told you in confidence can be a gray area. If you feel you need guidance, talk to your supervisor.

When a patient's pain is too much to bear

There is a widespread practice of undermedicating pain in this country, partly the result of clinicians' fears of causing death.[8] And yet, aggressively managing the symptoms of a terminally ill patient is both legally and ethically justifiable if treatment is carried out in accordance with accepted standards of care.

The ANA's *Code for Nurses*, for example, states that nurses caring for dying patients may provide interventions to relieve symptoms " even when the interventions entail substantial risks of hastening death."[6]

While reluctance to adequately medicate is common, sometimes nurses will encounter the opposite problem. What should you do if the doctor of a terminally ill patient prescribes a dose that is so large you believe it will directly cause the patient's death?

First, validate your concerns by checking the patient's clinical condition, pain history, and dosage requirements. If you still have questions, raise them with the attending physician.

If that discussion does not dispel your doubts, go through your institution's chain of command. If you still believe that it is unsafe to administer the dose, do not do so. Promptly inform the patient's attending physician and your supervisor that you will not carry out this order and explain the reason why.

Document all your contacts regarding the medication order in the patient's chart. Afterward, fill out an incident report or write a memo about the episode, stating just the facts. Give a copy to your supervisor and keep one for yourself.

Most patients find it very difficult to talk about dying. So do most health care professionals. As a result, we miss windows of opportunity to engage patients in discussions that could improve the end of life.

The nurse's role now: comfort, inform, advocate

Contrary to popular belief, discussing suicidal thoughts doesn't make suicide more likely. It may even reduce the chances of it happening.[4] When you care for a terminally ill patient—even before he has reached the end stage of his disease—let him know that you or an appropriate staff member are available to talk and answer questions.

Make sure he understands that he cannot be forced to have intrusive treatments. Educate him so he can make informed decisions about his care, and educate his family, if appropriate. Identify community support groups.

Advocate for your patient if he has made out an advance directive but the wishes expressed in it are not being followed.

Be an advocate within your institution for better pain assessment and control, too.

If we truly want to meet patients' end-of-life needs, we can't afford to wait until their final moments to do it.

REFERENCES

1. Washington v. Glucksberg, 79 F.3d 790 (9th Cir.1996).
2. Quill v. Vacco, 80 F.3d 716 (2nd Cir. 1996).
3. Greve, P. (1994). Has the PSDA made a difference? RN, 57(2), 59.
4. American Nurses Association. (1994). Position statement on assisted suicide. Washington, DC: Author.
5. American Nurses Association. (1994). Position statement on active euthanasia. Washington, DC: Author.
6. American Nurses Association. (1985). Code for nurses with interpretive statements. Kansas City, MO: Author.
7. Michigan Nurses Association. (1994). MNA Human Rights/Ethics Committee position statement on assisted voluntary self-termination. Okemos, MI: Author.
8. Solomon, M. Z., O'Donnell, L., et al. (1993). Decisions near the end of life: Professional views on life-sustaining treatments. Am. J. Public Health, 83(1), 14.

Malpractice Coverage

Should you have your own malpractice policy?

Worried about being sued? Buying your own malpractice coverage is an economical and effective way to ease your anxiety.

"**I**f I take out an individual malpractice policy, I'll increase my chances of being sued." Attorneys who present nursing seminars often hear that comment when they address a group of RNs. When they point out that having liability insurance does not invite lawsuits, their audience is often surprised.

In fact, whether you get sued has nothing to do with whether you have insurance. Attorneys and the patients they represent have no way of knowing if you have your own policy, or the extent of your coverage, until after they file charges.

Although a lot of nurses get by without their own insurance, nursing organizations do not recommend it. The reason: While it will not keep you from being sued, an individual policy lifts most of the financial burden and much of the fear of a lawsuit off your shoulders.

A standard policy costs a little over $100 a year, and obligates the insurance company to defend you and pay a verdict or settlement, should the need arise. Doing without it, says the ANA, is risky.[1] Having your own policy also fulfills what proponents view as your professional responsibility: It assures that there's a financial remedy available to anyone who's harmed as a result of your error or negligence.[2]

Only you, however, have the ability to decide whether or not your on-the-job insurance policy covers all of your malpractice insurance needs.

Why might an employer's coverage not be enough

Here are some key points to consider as you make your decision:

Your specialty. Although statistics are scarce, studies suggest that RNs who are in OB/GYN, intensive care, and med/surg are more likely to be involved in lawsuits than those in community or occupational health, school nursing, geriatrics, psych, or administration.[3] If you're in a high-risk specialty, you may decide you need additional coverage.

Consider your nursing specialty, too, when you shop for an individual policy. Because many state laws extend the statute of limitations for minors to a year or two after they reach adulthood, OB and pediatric nurses often prefer occurrence insurance. Unlike a claims-made policy, which covers you only for claims filed while the policy is in effect, an occurrence policy covers you for incidents that take place during the policy period but may not result in legal action until years later.

Off-the-job activities. Your employer's insurance covers you for acts or omissions that occur in the course of your work. If you use your nursing skills outside the workplace—giving advice to a friend or neighbor, for example, or volunteering to do BP checks in your community—only your own malpractice policy will protect you.

On-the-job activities. Although it's rare, your employer's insurance carrier could refuse to defend you against an action at work if that action fell outside the scope of your job. In a pamphlet for nurses, The American Association of Nurse Attorneys cites the example of ED nurses who pump blood to increase patients' replacement rate despite a written institutional policy prohibiting RNs from doing so.

To protect yourself and your patients and assure that everything you do on the job is covered by your employer's malpractice provider, be sure you're within the confines of existing policies and protocols. Individual coverage would extend to actions beyond the policies set forth by your employer as long as you act within the scope of your state's Nurse Practice Act.

Your employer's policy. Is your hospital self-insured, or does it have a commercial policy? If you don't know, talk to someone from risk management and read the fine print to find out.

Inquire, too, about what would happen to your coverage for on-the-job actions if your institution closed its doors or changed malpractice carriers, or you retired or went to work elsewhere. Employers with claims-made insurance should provide tail coverage to fill in any gaps created by a move from one insurance provider to another.

If you can't or don't want to rely on your employer or former employer to guarantee uninterrupted coverage, having your own policy could provide it.

Keep in mind, too, that an insurance company that provides your hospital's coverage might feel more allegiance to the hospital than to you. In most legal claims, your interests and the interests of your hospital will be similar. But there could be exceptions. If another employee with more clout pointed the finger at you, for example, having an individual liability policy assures you that someone will be working strictly for you.

Your assets and state laws. Although most cases are settled within the limits of insurance policies, it is possible for a verdict to exceed them. How much you stand to lose if you're sued and do not have adequate insurance depends on your financial resources and the laws in your state.

In some states, jointly owned money or property cannot be used to satisfy a settlement or award in a lawsuit against only one of the parties. In others, only resources owned jointly by spouses are exempt, while some states do not extend legal protection to personal assets at all.

If you're a public health employee, see if your state provides immunity for work-related activities. If so, you may feel little need for additional coverage. In all states, if you work for a federal facility, you're exempt from lawsuits related to your job.

Even here, however, there are exceptions to keep in mind: A public employee can be sued, of course, for an act outside the scope of employment. There may be instances, too, where you'd need the resources to mount a defense based on your immunity status.

Other laws that you must consider: Some states put a cap, or limit, on the amount an individual defendant or institution can be held liable for. If your state has such a cap in place, your already slight chance of losing all your assets becomes even slimmer. Some experts suggest, however, that you have a greater likelihood of being sued by plaintiffs who attempt to circumvent the cap by naming multiple defendants.

What about overlap

Soon after purchasing individual coverage, nurses ask: "If I'm involved in a lawsuit at work, will my policy or my hospital's policy cover me?" The answer depends on the policies and the circumstances. So ask questions, and read the fine print.

Often, one insurer identifies itself as your primary carrier. The other policy may have a clause stating that it's secondary, or excess, if other valid coverage exists. In that case, the secondary carrier—which could be either your employer's insurer or the one you secure on your own—would contribute only if a judgment exceeded the limits of the primary policy.

If neither policy defines itself as your primary or secondary carrier, the two may prorate the costs of your defense and any awards assessed.

Any confusion that comes from having your own insurance and your employer's coverage is no reason not to have both. To avoid complications, request clarification of both policies prior to any accident or incident. Then, if you are involved in an action that results in a lawsuit—or that you reasonably expect to result in a lawsuit—notify both providers. Be sure that each is aware of your coverage with the other.

What's expected of you? What can you expect?

Your obligation to an insurance provider begins when you first apply for coverage. You must answer all questions completely and honestly, whether they have to do with previous legal action, criminal record, history of substance abuse, or sanctions on your nursing license. Failure to tell the truth could invalidate the policy.

Should you need legal help, you must cooperate with your insurance carrier. Interfering with your defense, as by lying to the attorney who represents you or attempting to tamper with the medical records, would give your insurer grounds to refuse to represent you.

It's unlikely for any malpractice policy, whether it's employer-paid or your own, to cover you against criminal charges or administrative or disciplinary actions by the state Board of Nursing. For the civil liability claims that such policies do cover, however, having malpractice insurance gives you certain rights.

You have the right to legal defense, of course. But it is your insurer, not you, who selects the attorney who represents you.

If you believe you're not getting proper legal advice or think your employer's insurer is not working on your behalf, you also have the right to request other representation. But don't expect to be allowed to choose your own attorney or to have the final say about whether or when to settle. Having insurance also allows you to shift the financial burden of compensating an injured patient to your insurance company.

When a case is settled or a judgment awarded, malpractice insurers are required by law to report the action to the National Practitioner Data Bank. Launched in an attempt to track incompetent health care workers and reduce the incidence of malpractice, the data bank records the name of the individual in whose name the payment was made, the amount of the payment, and a description of the case. Hospital administrators must check the data bank before hiring or granting admitting privileges to any physician. They may check the data bank before hiring nurses, but are not required to do so.

What can you do to protect yourself? Be certain to get a copy of any report that is submitted to the National Practitioner Data Bank under your name. And, if you worry excessively about being sued, purchase an individual malpractice insurance policy to protect you.

REFERENCES

1. Think twice about relying on employer liability coverage. (1993, March). The American Nurse, 35.
2. The American Association of Nurse Attorneys. (1989). Demonstrating financial responsibility for nursing practice. Baltimore: Author.
3. Northrop, C. (1986). Nursing actions in litigation. Risk Management and Quality Assurance: Issues and Interactions 24. Chicago: Joint Commission on the Accreditation of Healthcare Organizations.

Appendices

How to contact your state nursing board

For application forms and answers to your questions about fees, licensing regulations, and continuing education requirements, contact the nursing board in the state where you plan to work.

Alabama
Board of Nursing, RSA Plaza,
Suite 250, 770 Washington Ave.,
P.O. Box 303900 Montgomery, AL 36130
(334) 242-4060

Alaska
Board of Nursing,
Division of Occupational Licensing,
Frontier Building, 3601 C St.,
Suite 722, Anchorage, AK 99503
(907) 269-8160

Arizona
State Board of Nursing,
1651 E. Morten Ave., Suite 150,
Phoenix, AZ 85020
(602) 255-5092

Arkansas
State Board of Nursing,
Suite 800, University Tower Building,
1123 S. University Ave.,
Little Rock, AR 72204
(501) 686-2700

California
Board of Registered Nursing,
P.O. Box 944210,
Sacramento, CA 94244-2100
(916) 322-3350

Colorado
State Board of Nursing,
1560 Broadway, Suite 670,
Denver, CO 80202
(303) 894-2430

Connecticut
Dept. Of Public Health,
Nurse Licensure, 410 Capitol Ave.
MS#12APP, PO Box 340308
Hartford, CT 06134
(860) 509-7570

Delaware
Board of Nursing,
Cannon Building, Suite 203,
P.O. Box 1401, Dover, DE 19903
(302) 739-4522, ext. 217

District of Columbia

Board of Nursing,
614 H St. N.W., Room 904,
Washington, DC 20001
(202) 727-7454

Florida

Board of Nursing,
4080 Woodcock Dr., Suite 202
Jacksonville, FL 32207
(904) 858-6940

Georgia

Board of Nursing,
166 Pryor St. S.W., Atlanta, GA 30303
(404) 656-3943

Hawaii

Board of Nursing, Box 3469,
Honolulu, HI 96801
(808) 586-3000

Idaho

State Board of Nursing,
P.O. Box 83720,
Boise, ID 83720-0061
(208) 334-3110

Illinois

Department of Professional Regulation,
320 W. Washington St., 3rd Floor,
Springfield, IL 62786
(217) 782-8556

Indiana

State Board of Nursing,
Indiana Government Center South,
402 W. Washington St., Room 041,
Indianapolis, IN 46204
(317) 232-1105

Iowa

Board of Nursing,
State Capitol Complex,
1223 E. Court Ave.,
Des Moines, IA 50319
(515) 281-3256

Kansas

State Board of Nursing,
Landon State Office Building,
900 S.W. Jackson, Suite 551-S,
Topeka, KS 66612-1230
(913) 296-4929

Kentucky

Board of Nursing,
312 Whittington Pkwy.,
Suite 300, Louisville, KY 41222-5172
(502) 329-7000

Louisiana

State Board of Nursing,
3510 N. Causeway Blvd., Suite 501,
Metarie, LA 70002
(504) 838-5332

Maine

State Board of Nursing,
24 Stone St.,
158 State House Station,
Augusta, ME 04333-0158
(207) 287-1183

Maryland

Board of Nursing,
4140 Patterson Ave.,
Baltimore, MD 21215
(410) 764-5124

Massachusetts

Board of Registration in Nursing,
100 Cambridge St., Room 1519,
Boston, MA 02202
(617) 727-9961

Michigan

Board of Nursing,
Dept. of Consumer & Industry
Services, Office of Health Services,
611 W. Ottawa, Box 30670,
Lansing, MI 48909
(517) 335-0918

Minnesota
Board of Nursing,
2829 University Ave. SE,
Minneapolis, MN 55414
(612) 617-2270

Mississippi
Board of Nursing,
239 N. Lamar St., Suite 401,
Jackson, MS 39201
(601) 359-6170

Missouri
State Board of Nursing,
P.O. Box 656,
Jefferson City, MO 65102
(573) 751-0681

Montana
Board of Nursing,
111 N. Jackson, Arcade Building,
P.O. Box 200513,
Helena, MT 59620-0513
(406) 444-2071

Nebraska
Board of Nursing,
Department of Health,
Professional & Occupational
Licensure Division, P.O. Box 95007,
Lincoln, NE 68509
(402) 471-0317

Nevada
Board of Nursing,
P.O. Box 46886,
Las Vegas, NV 89114
(702) 739-1575

New Hampshire
Board of Nursing,
Health and Welfare Building,
6 Hazen Drive,
Concord, NH 03301-6527
(603) 271-2323

New Jersey
Board of Nursing,
P.O. Box 45010, Newark, NJ 07101
(201) 504-6430

New Mexico
Board of Nursing,
4206 Louisiana NE, Suite A,
Albuquerque, NM 87109
(505) 841-8340

New York
State Education Department,
Division of Professional Licensing
Services, Cultural Education Center,
Empire State Plaza,
Albany, NY 12230
(518) 474-3817

North Carolina
Board of Nursing,
P.O. Box 2129,
Raleigh, NC 27602
(919) 782-3211

North Dakota
Board of Nursing,
Suite 504, 919 S. 7th St.,
Bismarck, ND 58504
(701) 328-9777

Ohio
Board of Nursing,
77 S. High St., 17th Floor,
Columbus, OH 43266-0316
(614) 466-3947

Oklahoma
Board of Nursing,
2915 N. Classen Blvd., Suite 524,
Oklahoma City, OK 73106
(405) 525-2076

Oregon
State Board of Nursing,
Suite 465, 800 N.E. Oregon St.,
Portland, OR 97232
(503) 731-4745

Pennsylvania
State Board of Nursing,
Department of State, Box 2649,
Harrisburg, PA 17105-2649
(717) 783-7142

Puerto Rico
Office of Regulations and
Certification of Health Professionals,
ATTN: Board of Nurse Examiners,
Call Box 10200,
San Juan, PR 00908
(787) 725-8161

Rhode Island
Board of Nurse Registration and
Nursing Education,
3 Capitol Hill, Room 104,
Providence, RI 02908
(401) 277-2827

South Carolina
State Board of Nursing,
P.O. Box 12367,
Columbia, SC 29211
(803) 869-4523

South Dakota
Board of Nursing,
3307 S. Lincoln Ave.,
Sioux Falls, SD 57105-5224
(605) 367-5940

Tennessee
Board of Nursing,
1st Floor, Cordell Hull Bldg.
425 5th Ave. North,
Nashville, TN 37247-1010
(615) 532-5166

Texas
Board of Nurse Examiners,
PO Box 430, Austin, TX 78767
(512) 305-7400

Utah
Division of Occupational and
Professional Licensing,
Board of Nursing,
160 E. 300 South, P.O. Box 146741,
Salt Lake City, UT 84114
(801) 530-6628

Vermont
Board of Nursing,
109 State St.,
Montpelier, VT 05609-1106
(802) 828-2396

Virginnia
Board of Nursing,
Department of Health Professions,
6606 West Broad St., 4th floor,
Richmond, VA 23230-1717
(804) 662-9909

Washington
State Nursing Care Quality
Assurance Commission,
1300 Quince St., P.O. Box 47864,
Olympia, WA 98504-7864
(360) 753-2686

West Virginia
Board of Examiners for
Registered Profesional Nurses,
101 Dee Dr.,
Charleston, WV 25311-1620
(304) 558-3596

Wisconsin
Bureau of Health Service Professions,
Box 8935, Madison, WI 53708-8935
(608) 266-0145

Wyoming
Board of Nursing,
2020 Carey Ave., Suite 110,
Cheyenne, WY 82002
(307) 777-7601

Appendix Two:

Standards of clinical nursing practice

The American Nurses Association established standards of clinical nursing practice to serve as guidelines for determining good nursing care. They are divided into two parts: standards of care and standards of professional performance. Generally, it is these standards to which nurses will be held by the legal system.

Standards of care

Standard I: Assessment

The nurse collects patient health data.

MEASUREMENT CRITERIA — SUMMARY
The patient's immediate condition or needs determines the priority the nurse sets on data collection. The nurse will use appropriate assessment techniques and will involve the patient, family members, and health care providers in the process when appropriate. Collecting data is a systematic and ongoing process and the data must be documented in retrievable form.

Standard II: Diagnosis

The nurse analyzes the assessment data in determining diagnoses.

MEASUREMENT CRITERIA — SUMMARY
Nursing diagnoses are derived from the assessment data, validated with those from whom the data was obtained, and documented so as to facilitate determining outcomes and planning care.

Standard III: Outcome identification

The nurse identifies expected outcomes individualized to the patient.

MEASUREMENT CRITERIA — SUMMARY
Outcomes are determined by the diagnoses and documented as measurable goals. They should be determined in consultation with the patient and other health care providers, when possible. Outcomes should be realistic and attainable given the patient's capabilities and the resources available. They should include a time estimate and take continuity of care into consideration.

Standard IV: Planning

The nurse develops a plan of care that prescribes interventions to attain expected outcomes.

MEASUREMENT CRITERIA — SUMMARY
The care plan must be individualized, developed in consultation with the patient, family members, and health care providers, and reflect current nursing practice. It must be documented and provide for continuity of care.

Standard V: Implementation

The nurse implements the interventions identified in the plan of care.

MEASUREMENT CRITERIA — SUMMARY
Nursing interventions should be consistent with the plan of care, be implemented safely, and be appropriately documented.

Standard VI: Evaluation

The nurse evaluates the patient's progress toward attainment of outcomes.

MEASUREMENT CRITERIA — SUMMARY
Evaluation must be systematic, ongoing, and documented. Documentation must include the patient's responses to the interventions. Effectiveness of interventions is evaluated based on the outcomes and is used to revise, if necessary, diagnoses, outcomes, and the plan or care.

Standards of professional performance

Standard I: Quality of Care

The nurse systematically evaluates the quality and effectiveness of nursing practice.

MEASUREMENT CRITERIA — SUMMARY
Nurses are expected to study and attempt to improve the quality of nursing care throughout the health care delivery system in a manner consistent with his or her position, education, and practice environment. Such activities include collecting and analyzing quality data, making recommendations to improve nursing practice or patient outcomes, and, if appropriate, developing policies and procedures to assure quality patient care.

Standard II: Performance appraisal

The nurse systematically evaluates her own nursing practice in relation to professional practice standards and relevant statutes and regulations.

MEASUREMENT CRITERIA — SUMMARY
Nurses should evaluate their own performance regularly, looking at strengths as well as areas that need development, seek

constructive feedback from others, and provide it to others when appropriate. Individuals are expected to act on the recommendations made during performance appraisals.

Standard III: Education

The nurse acquires and maintains current knowledge in nursing practice.

MEASUREMENT CRITERIA — SUMMARY
Continuing education in both clinical and professional areas appropriate to the practice environment are essential to the nurse. He or she must maintain clinical skills.

Standard IV: Collegiality

The nurse contributes to the professional development of peers, colleagues, and others.

MEASUREMENT CRITERIA — SUMMARY
A nurse must share knowledge and skills with colleagues, give constructive feedback to peers, and provide appropriate help in clinical education of nursing students.

Standard V: Ethics

The nurse's decisions and actions on behalf of patients are determined in an ethical manner.

MEASUREMENT CRITERIA — SUMMARY
A nurse's practice must be guided by the Code for Nurses. He or she must maintain patient confidentiality, act as a patient advocate preserving patient rights, care for patients in a nonjudgmental and nondiscriminatory manner sensitive to patient diversity. The nurse delivers care in a manner that preserves and protects patient autonomy, dignity, and rights. If he or she is unsure of the correct ethical course, he or she should seek help in determining it.

Standard VI: Collaboration

The nurse collaborates with the patient, family members, and health care providers regarding patient care and nursing's role in the provision of care.

MEASUREMENT CRITERIA — SUMMARY
All parties listed above should be recognized as part of the decision-making process regarding the patient's care and consulted with as appropriate. Referrals, including provisions for continuity of care, should be made as needed.

Standard VII: Research

The nurse uses research findings in practice.

MEASUREMENT CRITERIA — SUMMARY
Nursing interventions should be substantiated by research and nurses should participate in research activities as appropriate to the individual's position, education, and practice environment.

Standard VIII: Resource utilization

The nurse considers factors related to safety, effectiveness, and cost in planning and delivering patient care.

MEASUREMENT CRITERIA — SUMMARY
Factors related to safety, effectiveness, and cost must be considered when choosing between two or more practice options that would result in the same expected patient outcome. The nurse must assign tasks or delegate care based on patient needs and the knowledge and skills of the provider selected. The nurse should also be a resource for the patient and partner in securing appropriate services to address health-related needs.

The Standards of Clinical Practice are reprinted with permission of the American Nurses Association. Summaries of the Measurement Criteria have been adapted from those published by the ANA.

Standards of advanced practice registered nursing

As the scope of nursing practice grows, the American Nurses Association recognized a need for a separate set of standards for advanced practice nurses. These were published in 1996.

Standards of care

Standard I: Assessment

The advanced practice registered nurse collects comprehensive client health data.

MEASUREMENT CRITERIA — SUMMARY
Assessment should be research based and arrived at using appropriate diagnostic tests and procedures.

Standard II: Diagnosis

The advanced practice registered nurse critically analyzes the assessment data in determining diagnoses.

MEASUREMENT CRITERIA — SUMMARY
Complex clinical reasoning is applied to assessment data gathered during an interview and physical exam as well as diagnostic tests and procedures to make diagnoses and prioritize them. A differential diagnosis is made by systematically comparing clinical findings.

Standard III: Outcome identification

The advanced practice registered nurse identifies expected outcomes derived from the assessment data and diagnoses and individualizes expected outcomes with the client, and with the health care team when appropriate.

MEASUREMENT CRITERIA — SUMMARY
Expected outcomes are identified with consideration of the associated risk, benefits, and costs. They must be consistent with current scientific and clinical practice knowledge and must be modified based on changes in the client's health care status.

Standard IV: Planning

The advanced practice registered nurse develops a comprehensive plan of care that includes interventions and treatments to attain expected outcomes.

MEASUREMENT CRITERIA — SUMMARY
The plan of care describes assessment and diagnostic strategies and therapeutic interventions that reflect current knowledge, research, and practice. It reflects responsibilities of both nurse and client, and may include delegation of responsibilities to others. The plan of care should also address strategies for promotion and restoration of health and prevention of illness, injury, and disease through independent clinical decision-making and must be documented and modifiedd to provide direction to other members of the health care team.

Standard V: Implementation

The advanced practice registered nurse prescribes, orders, or implements interventions and treatments for the plan of care.

MEASUREMENT CRITERIA — SUMMARY
Interventions and treatments must be based on knowledge of

health care research, reflect a scientific basis and theory, and fall within the scope of advanced practice registered nursing.

Standard Va: Case Management/Coordination of Care

The advanced practice registered nurse provides comprehensive clinical coordination of care and case management.

MEASUREMENT CRITERIA — SUMMARY
Case management and clinical coordination of care are provided using sophisticated data synthesis with consideration of all the client's needs and the desired outcomes in order to provide integration of health care that is accessible, available, high quality, and cost-effective. Additional services and specialized care are negotiated with the client, appropriate systems, agencies, and providers.

Standard Vb: Consultation

The advanced practice registered nurse provides consultation to influence the plan of care for clients, enhance the abilities of others, and effect change in the system.

MEASUREMENT CRITERIA — SUMMARY
Consultation is based on theoretical frameworks and mutual respect, and defined role responsibility is established with the client. Consultation recommendations should be communicated in terms the client can understand and should involve the client in the decision-making, but it remains the responsibility of the client to implement recommendations.

Standard Vc: Health Promotion, Health Maintenance, and Health Teaching

The advanced practice registered nurse employs complex strategies, interventions, and teaching to promote, maintain, and improve health, and prevent illness and injury.

MEASUREMENT CRITERIA — SUMMARY

Health promotion and prevention strategies must be based on assessment of risks, learning theory, epidemiological principles, and the client's health beliefs and practices. Health promotion, maintenance, and teaching methods should be appropriate to the client's developmental level, learning needs, readiness and ability to learn, and the culture from which he comes.

Standard Vd: Prescriptive Authority and Treatment

The advanced practice registered nurse uses prescriptive authority, procedures, and treatment in accordance with state and federal laws and regulations to treat illness and improve functional health status or to provide preventive care.

MEASUREMENT CRITERIA — SUMMARY

Treatment interventions and procedures are based on current knowledge, practice, and research and are prescribed according to the client's health care needs. Procedures are done as indicated to deliver comprehensive care. Pharmacologic agents are prescribed based on a knowledge of pharmacological and physiological principles, on clincial indicators or on the client's status and needs, including the results of diagnostic and lab tests. Effects of pharmacologic and non-pharmacologic treatments are monitored and appropriate information about intended effects, potential adverse effects, costs, and alternative treatments and procedures is provided to the client.

Standard Ve: Referral

The advanced practice registered nurse identifies the need for additional care and makes referrals as needed.

MEASUREMENT CRITERIA — SUMMARY

As the primary health care provider, the advanced practice registered nurse implements recommendations from referral sources and refers directly to other providers based on client needs with consideration of benefits and costs.

Standard VI: Evaluation

The advanced practice registered nurse evaluates the client's progress in attaining expected outcomes.

MEASUREMENT CRITERIA — SUMMARY
Diagnoses and interventions are evaluated according to the client's attainment of the expected outcomes. The evaluation process is based on advanced knowledge, practice, and research, and results in revision or resolution of diagnoses, outcomes, and plan of care.

Standards of professional performance

Standard I: Quality of Care

The advanced practice registered nurse develops criteria for and evaluates the quality and effectiveness of advanced practice registered nursing.

MEASUREMENT CRITERIA — SUMMARY
The advanced practice registered nurse assumes a leadership role in establishing and monitoring standards of practice to improve client care, uses the results of quality of care activities to initiate changes throughout the health care system, participates in efforts to minimize costs and unnecessary duplication of testing or other diagnostic activities and to facilitate timely treatment of the client, analyzes factors related to safety, satisfaction, effectiveness, and cost/benefit options with the client, and other providers as appropriate. He or she also analyzes organizational systems for barriers that affect client health care and promotes changes as appropriate. Advanced practice registered nurses base their evaluations on current knowledge, practice, and research and seek professional certification when available.

Standard II: Performance appraisal

Advanced practice registered nurses continuously evaluate their own nursing practice in relation to professional practice standards and relevant statutes and regulation, and are acountable to the public and to the profession for providing competent clinical care.

MEASUREMENT CRITERIA
The advanced practice registered nurse must evaluate his or her own performance according to the standards of the profession, various regulatory bodies, and client outcomes, and must take action to improve practice, seeking feedback regarding practice and role performance from peers, professional colleagues, clients, and others.

Standard III: Education

The advanced practice registered nurse acquires and maintains current knowledge and skills in the area of specialty practice.

MEASUREMENT CRITERIA — SUMMARY
The advanced practice registered nurse uses current research to expand clinical knowledge, enhance performancce, and increase knowledge of professional issues. He or she seeks experiences and formal and independent learning activities to maintain and develop clinical and professional skills and knowledge.

Standard IV: Leadership

The advanced practice registered nurse serves as a leader and a role model for the professional development of peers, colleagues, and others.

MEASUREMENT CRITERIA — SUMMARY
To improve client care and foster growth of the profession, the advanced practice registered nurse contributes to the profession-al development of others, including students, using creativity and innovation. The advanced practice registered nurse also works to influence policy-making bodies to improve client care.

Standard V: Ethics

The advanced pratice registered nurse integrates ethical principles and norms in all areas of practice.

MEASUREMENT CRITERIA — SUMMARY
The advanced practice registered nurse maintains a therapeutic
and professional relationship with clients and defines the roles
of each party in the relationship, and informs the client of the
risks, benefits, and outcomes of health care regimens. He or she
contributes to resolving the ethical problems or dilemmas of
individuals or systems.

Standard VI: Interdisciplinary Process

The advanced practice registered nurse promotes an interdisciplinary process in providing client care.

MEASUREMENT CRITERIA — SUMMARY
The advanced practice registered nurse works with other disciplines
through education, consultation, management, technological
development, or research opportunities to enhance client care
and facilitates an interdisciplinary process with other members
of the health care team.

Standard VII: Research

The advanced practice registered nurse utilizes research to
discover, examine, and evaluate knowledge, theories, and creative
approaches to health care practice.

MEASUREMENT CRITERIA — SUMMARY
The advanced practice registered nurse critically evaluates
existing practice in light of current research findings, identifies
research questions in practice, and disseminates relevant
findings through practice, education, or consultation.

*The Standards of Advanced Practice Registered Nursing are reprinted with permission
of the American Nurses Association. Summaries of the Measurement Criteria have been
adapted from those published by the ANA.*

Code for Nurses

The American Nurses Association's Code for Nurses establishes principles of ethical nursing practice. Extensive interpretive statements (available through the ANA) expand each of the 11 principles set out below.

1. The nurse provides services with respect for human dignity and the uniqueness of the client, unrestricted by considerations of social or economic status, personal attributes, or the nature of health problems.

2. The nurse safeguards the client's right to privacy by judiciously protecting information of a confidential nature.

3. The nurse acts to safeguard the client and the public when health care and safety are affected by the incompetent, unethical, or illegal practice of any person.

4. The nurse assumes responsibility and accountability for individual nursing judgments and actions.

5. The nurse maintains competence in nursing.

6. The nurse exercises informed judgment and uses individual competence and qualifications as criteria in seeking consultation, accepting responsibilities, and delegating nursing activities to others.

7. The nurse participates in activities that contribute to the ongoing development of the profession's body of knowledge.

8. The nurse participates in the profession's efforts to implement and improve standards of nursing.

9. The nurse participates in the profession's efforts to establish and maintain conditions of employment conducive to high quality nursing care.

10. The nurse participates in the profession's effort to protect the public from misinformation and misrepresentation and to maintain the integrity of nursing.

11. The nurse collaborates with members of the health professions and other citizens in promoting community and national efforts to meet the health needs of the public.

Appendix Five:

How to contact your state nurses association

Here are the addresses, and telephone numbers of nurses associations in the United States and its territories. Association staff should be able to answer questions about the law in your state as it applies to nurses and to refer you to attorneys familiar with nurses' legal needs.

Alabama State Nurses' Association
360 N. Hull St.
Montgomery, AL 36104-3658
(205) 262-8321

Alaska Nurses Association
237 E. Third Ave., Suite 3
Anchorage, AK 99501
(907) 274-0827

Arizona Nurses Association
1850 E. Southern Ave., Suite 1
Tempe, AZ 85282-5832
(602) 831-0404

Arkansas Nurses' Association
117 S. Cedar St.
Little Rock, AR 72205
(501) 664-5853

California Nurses Association
1145 Market St., Suite 1100
San Francisco, CA 94103
(415) 864-4141

Colorado Nurses' Association
5453 E. Evans Place
Denver, CO 80222
(303) 757-7483 Ext. 3

Connecticut Nurses' Association
Meritech Business Park
377 Research Parkway, Suite 2D
Meridan, CT 06450
(203) 238-1207

**Delaware Nurses'
Association**
2634 Capitol Trail, Suite A
Newark, DE 19711
(302) 368-2333

**District of Columbia
Nurses' Association**
5100 Wisconsin Ave., N.W., Suite 306
Washington, DC 20016
(202) 244-2705

Florida Nurses Association
P.O. Box 536985
Orlando, FL 32853-6985
(407) 896-3261

Georgia Nurses Association
1362 W. Peachtree St., N.W.
Atlanta, GA 30309
(404) 876-4624

Guam Nurses' Association
P.O. Box 3134
Agana, Guam 96910
011 (671) 649-4930

Hawaii Nurses' Association
677 Ala Moana Blvd., #301
Honolulu, HI 96813
(808) 531-1628

Idaho Nurses Association
200 N. Fourth St., Suite 20
Boise, ID 83702-6001
(208) 345-0500

Illinois Nurses Association
200 S. Wacker, Suite 2200
Chicago, IL 60606
(312) 360-2300

**Indiana State Nurses'
Association**
2915 N. High School Road
Indianapolis, IN 46224-2969
(317) 299-4575

Iowa Nurses' Association
1501 42nd St., Suite 471
West Des Moines, IA 50266
(515) 225-0495

**Kansas State Nurses
Association**
700 S.W. Jackson, Suite 601
Topeka, KS 66603-3731
(913) 233-8638

**Kentucky Nurses
Association**
1400 South First St.
Louisville, KY 40201
(502) 637-2546

**Louisiana State Nurses
Association**
712 Transcontinental Dr.
Metairie, LA 70001
(504) 889-1030

**Maine State Nurses'
Association**
283 Water St.
P.O. Box 2240
Augusta, ME 04338-2240
(207) 622-1057

**Maryland Nurses
Association**
849 International Dr.
Airport Square 21, Suite 255
Linthicum, MD 21090
(410) 859-3000

**Massachusetts Nurses
Association**
340 Turnpike St.
Canton, MA 02021
(617) 821-4625

Michigan Nurses Association
2310 Jolly Oak Rd.
Okemos, MI 48864
(517) 349-5640

Minnesota Nurses Association
1295 Bandanna Blvd.. N., Suite 140
St. Paul, MN 55108
(612) 646-4807

Mississippi Nurses' Association
135 Bounds St., Suite 100
Jackson, MS 39206
(601) 982-9182

Missouri Nurses Association
206 E. Dunlkin St.
Jefferson City, MO 65102-0325
(314) 636-4623

Montana Nurses' Association
104 Broadway, Suite G-2
Helena, MT 59601
(406) 442-6710

Nebraska Nurses' Association
941 "O" St., Suite 707-711
Lincoln, NE 68508
(402) 475-3859

Nevada Nurses' Association
3660 Baker Lane, Suite 104
Reno, NV 89509
(702) 825-3555

New Hampshire Nurses' Association
48 West St.
Concord, NH 03301
(603) 225-3783

New Jersey State Nurses Association
320 W. State St.
Trenton, NJ 08618
(609) 392-4884

New Mexico Nurses Association
909 Virginia N.E., Suite 101
Albuquerque, NM 87108
(505) 268-7744

New York State Nurses Association
46 Cornell Rd.
Latham, NY 12110
(518) 782-9400

North Carolina Nurses Association
103 Enterprise St.
Raleigh, NC 27605-2025
(919) 821-4250

North Dakota Nurses' Association
212 N. Fourth St.
Bismarck, ND 58501
(701) 223-1385

Ohio Nurses Association
4000 E. Main St.
Columbus, OH 43213-2950
(614) 237-5414

Oklahoma Nurses Association
6414 N. Santa Fe, Suite A
Oklahoma City, OK 73116
(405) 840-3476

Oregon Nurses Association
9600 S.W. Oak, Suite 550
Portland, OR 97223
(503) 293-0011

Pennsylvania Nurses Association
2578 Interstate Dr.
Harrisburg, PA 17110
(717) 657-1222

Rhode Island State Nurses' Association
300 Ray Dr., Suite 5
Providence, RI 02906
(401) 421-9703

South Carolina Nurses' Association
1821 Gadsden St.
Columbia, SC 29201
(803) 252-4781

South Dakota Nurses' Association
1505 S. Minnesota, Suite 3
Sioux Falls, SD 57105
(605) 338-1401

Tennessee Nurses' Association
545 Mainstream Dr., Suite 405
Nashville, TN 37228-1207
(615) 254-0350

Texas Nurses Association
7600 Burnet Rd., Suite 440
Austin, TX 78757
(512) 452-0645

Utah Nurses' Association
455 East 400 South, Suite 402
Salt Lake City, UT 84111
(801) 322-3439

Vermont State Nurses' Association
Box 36 Champlain Mill, 1 Main St.
Winooski, VT 05404
(802) 655-7123

Virgin Islands Nurses' Association
P.O. Box 583
Christiansted, St. Croix 00821
(809) 773-2323 Ext. 119

Virginia Nurses' Association
7113 Three Chopt Rd., Suite 204
Richmond, VA 23226
(804) 282-1808

Washington State Nurses Association
2505 Second Ave., Suite 500
Seattle, WA 98121
(206) 443-9762

West Virginia Nurses Association
P.O. Box 1946
Charleston, WV 25327
(304) 342-1169

Wisconsin Nurses Association
6117 Monona Dr.
Madison, WI 53716
(608) 221-0383

Wyoming Nurses Association
Majestic Building, Room 305
1603 Capitol Ave.
Cheyenne, WY 82001
(307) 635-3955

AHA Patient's Bill of Rights

The American Hospital Association (AHA) first promulgated its Patient's Bill of Rights in the mid-'70s. Although it's not a binding document, many hospitals have adopted it as a guideline for patient care. It's often distributed as is to patients on admission or used as a model for an institution's own handout.

A patient's bill of rights

1. The patient has the right to considerate and respectful care.
2. The patient has the right to obtain from his doctor complete current information about his diagnosis, treatment, and prognosis in terms the patient can be reasonably expected to understand. When it is not medically advisable to give such information to the patient, it should be made available to an appropriate person in his behalf. He has the right to know, by name, the doctor responsible for coordinating his care.
3. The patient has the right to receive from his doctor information necessary to give informed consent prior to the start of any procedure or treatment. Except in emergencies, such information for informed consent should include but not necessarily be limited to the specific procedure or treatment, the medically significant risks involved, and the probable duration of incapacitation.

Where medically significant alternatives for care or treatment
exist, or when the patient requests information concerning
medical alternatives, the patient has the right to such information.
The patient has the right to know the name of the person
responsible for the procedures or treatment.

4. The patient has the right to refuse treatment to the
extent permitted by law and to be informed of the medical
consequences of his action.

5. The patient has the right to every consideration of his privacy
concerning his own medical care program. Case discussion,
consultation, examination, and treatment are confidential and
should be conducted discreetly. Those not directly involved in
his care must have the permission of the patient to be present.

6. The patient has the right to expect that all communications
and records pertaining to his care should be treated as
confidential.

7. The patient has the right to expect that within its capacity
a hospital must make reasonable response to the request of a
patient for services. The hospital must provide evaluation, service,
or referral as indicated by the urgency of the case. When
medically permissible, a patient may be transferred to another
facility only after he has received complete information and
explanation concerning the needs for and alternatives to such a
transfer. The institution to which the patient is to be transferred
must first have accepted the patient for transfer.

8. The patient has the right to obtain information as to any
relationship of his hospital to other health care and educational
institutions insofar as his care is concerned. The patient has the
right to obtain information as to the existence of any professional
relationships among individuals, by name, who are treating him.

9. The patient has the right to be advised if the hospital
proposes to engage in or perform human experimentation
affecting his care or treatment. The patient has the right to
refuse to participate in such research projects.

10. The patient has the right to expect reasonable continuity of care. He has the right to know in advance what appointment times and doctors are available and where. The patient has the right to expect that the hospital will provide a mechanism whereby he is informed by his doctor or a delegate of the doctor of the patient's continuing health care requirements following discharge.

11. The patient has the right to examine and receive an explanation of his bill, regardless of source of payment.

12. The patient has the right to know what hospital rules and regulations apply to his conduct as a patient.

Reprinted with permission of the
American Hospital Association,©1992.

ACLU Patient's Bill of Rights

Yet another statement of patient's rights was put together by the American Civil Liberties Union (ACLU). It gets much more specific than the AHA's document and focuses on the patient advocate role within the hospital, one that, for the most part didn't exist when the AHA first put its document together.

Preamble

As you enter this health care facility, it is our duty to remind you that your health care is a cooperative effort between you as a patient and the doctors and hospital staff. During your stay a patient's rights advocate will be available to you. The duty of the advocate is to assist you in all the decisions you must make and in all situations in which your health and welfare are at stake. The advocate's first responsibility is to help you understand the role of all who will be working with you, and to help you understand what your rights as a patient are. Your advocate can be reached at any time of the day by dialing _____.
The following is a list of your rights as a patient. Your advocate's duty is to see to it that you are afforded these rights. You should call your advocate whenever you have any questions or concerns about any of these rights.

Patient rights

■ The patient has a legal right to informed participation in all decisions involving his health care program.

■ We recognize the right of all potential patients to know what research and experimental protocols are being used in our facility and what alternatives are available in the community.

■ The patient has a legal right to privacy regarding the source of payment for treatment and care. This right includes access to the highest degree of care without regard to the source of payment for that treatment and care.

■ We recognize the right of a potential patient to complete and accurate information concerning medical care and procedures.

■ The patient has a legal right to prompt attention, especially in an emergency situation.

■ The patient has a legal right to a clear, concise explanation in layperson's terms of all proposed procedures, including the possibilities of any risk of mortality or serious side effects, problems related to recuperation, and probability of success, and will not be subjected to any procedure without his voluntary, competent, and understanding consent. The specifics of such consent shall be set out in a written consent form, signed by the patient.

■ The patient has a legal right to a clear, complete, and accurate evaluation of his condition and prognosis without treatment before being asked to consent to any test or procedure.

■ We recognize the right of the patient to know the identity and professional status of all those providing service. All personnel have been instructed to introduce themselves, state their status, and explain their role in the health care of the patient. Part of this right is the right of the patient to know the identity of the doctor responsible for his care.

■ We recognize the right of any patient who does not speak English to have access to an interpreter.

■ The patient has a right to all the information contained in his medical record while in the health care facility, and to examine the record on request.

■ We recognize the right of a patient to discuss his condition with a consultant specialist, at the patient's request and expense.

■ The patient has a legal right not to have any test or procedure, designed for educational purposes rather than his direct personal benefit, performed on him.

■ The patient has a legal right to refuse any particular drug, test, procedure, or treatment.

■ The patient has a legal right to privacy of both person and information with respect to the hospital staff, other doctors, residents, interns and medical students, researchers, nurses, other hospital personnel, and other patients.

■ We recognize the patient's right of access to people outside the health care facility by means of visitors and the telephone. Parents may stay with their children and relatives with terminally ill patients 24 hours a day.

■ The patient has a legal right to leave the health care facility regardless of his physical condition or financial status, although the patient may be requested to sign a release stating that he is leaving against the medical judgment of his doctor or the hospital.

■ The patient has a right not to be transferred to another facility unless he has received a complete explanation of the desirability of and need for the transfer. If the patient does not agree to transfer, the patient has the right to a consultant's opinion on the desirability of transfer.

■ A patient has a right to be notified of his impending discharge at least one day before it is accomplished, to insist on a consultation by an expert on the desirability of discharge, and to have a person of the patient's choice notified in advance.

■ The patient has a right, regardless of the source of payment, to examine and receive an itemized and detailed explanation of the total bill for services rendered in the facility.

■ The patient has a right to competent counseling from the hospital staff to help in obtaining financial assistance from public or private sources to meet the expense of services received in the institution.

■ The patient has a right to timely prior notice of the termination of his eligibility for reimbursement by any third-party payer for the expense of hospital care.

■ At the termination of his stay at the health care facility we recognize the right of a patient to a complete copy of the information contained in his medical record.

■ We recognize the right of all patients to have 24-hour-a-day access to a patient's rights advocate, who may act on behalf of the patient to assert or protect the rights set out in this document.

Reprinted with permission of the American Civil Liberties Union.

Index

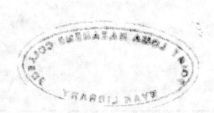